"I love this book, all of it. The polished essays and the interviews with birth workers dare to take on the deepest questions of human existence."
—Carol Downer, cofounder of the Feminist Women's Heath Centers of California and author of *A Woman's Book of Choices*

"This volume provides theoretically rich, practical tools for birth workers and other care workers to collectively and effectively fight capitalism and the many intersecting processes of oppression that accompany it. *Birth Work as Care Work* forcefully and joyfully reminds us that the personal is political, a lesson we need now more than ever."
—Adrienne Pine, author of *Working Hard, Drinking Hard: On Violence and Survival in Honduras*

"This book places the doula—as a caring birth activist—at the heart of reproductive care work in our modern society. Doula, a new name for an ancient traditional role, reappears today as women daring to reclaim their power through birthing and caring for their children."
—Valérie Dupin, cofounder and cochair of the Association Doulas de France

"All we are doing in this world is living and dying, creating and destroying. We generate new life in our children and in our ideas. Becoming a birth supporter, getting to be an attendant to the miracle of childbirth, has transformed my social justice work. Our visions for justice are what we are birthing in this world. Learning to listen, learning to trust the body and the people, and learning to breathe will transform our movement work. *Birth Work as Care Work* demonstrates these lessons through showing us ways we can learn together to sup
—Adrienne Brown, coedit
Fiction Stories from S

T0125826

"Alana Apfel is an artist and a robust one. Weaving the logic behind birth, care, and reproduction together, *Birth Work as Care Work* documents how caregivers and communities are marginalized in society on a daily basis whilst working to sustain themselves and ironically, to sustain life itself. Her thesis seeks to put the human back into being."
—Chitra Subramaniam, editor in chief of *The News Minute*

"Alana Apfel's nuanced *Birth Work as Care Work* moves us away from a 'choice' narrative to an understanding of the need for justice based on a politics of care work. The book will be a necessary movement builder because of the honesty and complexity of the wisdom spoken."
—Susan M. Reverby, professor of Women's and Gender Studies, Wellesley College

"Against an infinity of individualizing self-help books on birth and mothering, this anthology outlines a politics of birth through multiple voices. Birth is a central moment in the lives of collectives, involving a variety of participants and possibilities for change. Breaking with the invisibility and undervaluing of the reproductive sphere, this book shows what collective life and social movements can learn from birth in relation to labour, care work, community, and mothering."
—Manuela Zechner, the Nanopolitics Group

"Whether in the hospital, at home, or in the jail, doulas lovingly support the mom throughout the entire experience and into the postpartum period. *Birth Work as Care Work* powerfully demonstrates this through testimonies of birth experiences and in discussion of diverse aspects of the work. A must read."
— Maddy Oden, doula and executive director of the Tatia Oden French Memorial Foundation

Birth Work as Care Work

K A I R O S

In ancient Greek philosophy, *kairos* signifies the right time or the "moment of transition." We believe that we live in such a transitional period. The most important task of social science in time of transformation is to transform itself into a force of liberation. Kairos, an editorial imprint of the Anthropology and Social Change department housed in the California Institute of Integral Studies, publishes groundbreaking works in critical social sciences, including anthropology, sociology, geography, theory of education, political ecology, political theory, and history.

Series editor: Andrej Grubačić

Kairos books:

In, Against, and Beyond Capitalism: The San Francisco Lectures by John Holloway

Anthropocene or Capitalocene? Nature, History, and the Crisis of Capitalism edited by Jason W. Moore

Birth Work as Care Work: Stories from Activist Birth Communities by Alana Apfel

Wrapped in the Flag of Israel: Mizrahi Single Mothers, Israeli Ultranationalism, and Bureaucratic Torture by Smadar Lavie

We Are the Crisis of Capital: A John Holloway Reader by John Holloway

Birth Work as Care Work

Stories from Activist Birth Communities

Alana Apfel

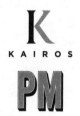

KAIROS

PM

Birth Work as Care Work: Stories from Activist Birth Communities
Alana Apfel
© 2016 PM Press.

All rights reserved. No part of this book may be transmitted by any
means without permission in writing from the publisher.

ISBN: 978-1-62963-151-6
Library of Congress Control Number: 2016930964

Cover by John Yates / www.stealworks.com
Interior design by briandesign

10 9 8 7 6 5 4 3 2 1

PM Press
PO Box 23912
Oakland, CA 94623
www.pmpress.org

Printed in the USA

Contents

For my mother, who gave me birth

Acknowledgments

This book was made possible through the support and contribution of many incredible people. Thank you to my teacher and friend Andrej Grubačić for putting an early version of this book forward for publication. Thank you to everyone from PM Press who helped make this happen: Ramsey Kanaan, Romy Ruukel, Gregory Nipper, John Yates, Jonathan Rowland, Steven Stothard, and Camille Barbagallo, and to Brian Layng for the beautiful design work. Thank you to Loretta Ross, Silvia Federici, and Victoria Law for writing introductions to the book. What you have collectively brought to feminism and to liberatory political projects throughout the world is truly legendary. I am honored to collaborate with you all. A huge thank you to all the contributors who shared their story with me in interviews: Jodi Koumouitzes-Douvia, Kelly Gray, Laili Falatoonzadeh, Cynthea Denise, Yania Escobar, Molly Arthur, Jewel Buchanan-Boone, and Sophia Perez. Your collective dedication to birth and Reproductive Justice is unfailing and an inspiration for all involved in this struggle. A special thank you to Grace Saras, Joanna Morrison, Donae Snow, and Marina Cochran-Keith, whose births inspired the doula stories included in this book. You are warriors. Never forget it. Lastly, thank you to my father, Franklin Apfel, for your unwavering support, endless Skype conversations, and that dance move.

Foreword
Loretta J. Ross

I was terribly afraid to begin this piece on birth work. It took me a while to figure out why. My experience with birthing was probably the primary reason. I remember the trauma of my birthing experience when I was fifteen. I was pregnant because of incest, rape by a married cousin twelve years older than me. I had no choice about whether to have the baby because abortion was illegal and largely inaccessible in the 1960s. My mother stuck me in a home for unwed pregnant girls to hide me from the community. We jointly planned to give the baby up for adoption. The home was run by the Salvation Army, whose workers offered a bizarre combination of compassion and religious zealotry that blamed our pregnancies on our alleged immorality and our failure to sufficiently believe in Jesus. There was no space to talk about incest, child sexual abuse, or even the progress of our pregnancies in this setting. We woke up early every day to pray, clean the buildings, listen inattentively to a school tutor, and count the painfully slow minutes until we were liberated from this pseudo-prison by the labor pains of birth. For me, going into labor signaled liberation from confinement, returning to my family, and forgetting the horror of the entire pregnancy. It did not mean becoming a mother, because I had no intention of keeping the child of my rapist.

Until my son was born. The hospital nurses "accidentally" brought my son to me after his birth. I question whether it was an accident because the hospital policy was that children scheduled to be adopted were *not* to be brought to their mothers for nursing. Yet, my son was placed on my breast the next morning and all I could say was, "He's got my face . . . he's got my face" in wonder as the miracle of mother bonding overwhelmed all of my previous decisions about this little person suckling on me. So I decided to keep my son, and I have co-parented with my rapist for the past forty-seven years. I cannot overstate the impact of this decision on me and my son. While I dearly love my child, he has never received from me the unconditional love every child deserves because I had to love him despite the circumstances of his conception and birth. This type of unresolved trauma lingers in my DNA and affects my worldview, my relationships, and my physical being even now.

As if the circumstances of my pregnancy were not enough drama, I also endured some careless brutality in the birthing process itself. After about fourteen hours of labor, I was placed in a hospital prep room with another teenager also in labor. My pubic area was shaved and I was checked to see how far I had dilated. While waiting between contractions, I noticed some little bugs crawling on my bed. I am bug-phobic, so I quickly called the nurse who identified the bugs as lice crawling from my neighbor's bed. So in the middle of labor, I had to be fumigated. In fact, the entire ward had to be evacuated, and I think the extra work pissed off the nighttime staff because they were extremely mean to all of us after that. I often wonder what they did to that young girl from my room because I fear they punished her even more harshly.

The debugging pushed me over the edge. After another four hours of intense labor, I was screaming so loud from the combination of fear and pain that the hospital staff simply ignored me, the way that some mothers can ignore their children's tantrums. I didn't know what was happening to my body. No one had explained the process of pregnancy and delivery to me. Hell, no one had even told me about sex! Everything just seemed to happen without cause, without meaning. My mother did not come to the hospital. I'm not sure why, except that possibly the trauma of her own experiences with childhood sexual abuse probably lingered in her soul, and she couldn't stand to watch her daughter's pain that created resonances with her own unhealed grief. Alone and scared, I was a mindless screamer. Finally a doctor demanded that someone "knock this girl out" so he could get on with the delivery.

So I had what I later found out was called a "twilight delivery." I was unconscious and only woke up briefly when a nurse was pressing my stomach to push out afterbirth. I don't remember my son's delivery; his birth certificate says it happened at 4:19 on a Wednesday morning. Six hours later, I was fighting the adoption administrators for my right to keep him. That's when my mother finally showed up at the hospital to argue me out of my decision. So I subconsciously strove to forget my birthing trauma, as if I were self-administering a date-rape drug.

Twenty-five years later, in 1994, I was one of twelve African American women who created the Reproductive Justice framework, which emerged from our practices in the black feminist movement. We needed a way to move beyond the stymied pro-choice/anti-abortion debates, and we envisioned ourselves in the center of the lens when we defined what we deserved from the debates on reproductive politics. As African American women, we joined with the pro-choice movement to fight for the human right to not have children by using birth control, abortion, and abstinence. But as targets of strategies of eugenics and population control, we had to fight equally as hard for the human right to have the children we wanted, under the conditions we choose, such as the use of midwives and doulas. And finally, we had to fight for the right to parent our children in safe and healthy environments, because our children's lives are endlessly threatened in a myriad of ways that include police brutality, environmental toxins, out-of-control gun and rape cultures, and neoliberal capitalism, among the many forces too numerous to fully name here. We have to protect our children from the monstrous appetite of white supremacy.

Thus Reproductive Justice is the multivocality of black women's lives put into action, and emphasizes bodily autonomy, human dignity, and self-determination to counter the pathologizing of black women's bodies and decisions. Although Reproductive Justice was created by African American women, it does not only apply to black women. Every human being has an intersectional identity that deserves to be honored in order for them to achieve their full human rights. Intersectionality is the process; human rights are the goal. Reproductive Justice turns relationships of difference into politically powerful forces capable of destabilizing reproductive oppressions such as xenophobia, racism, sexism, transphobia, ageism, ableism, and homophobia. Reproductive Justice helps people process the trauma, disrespect, and abuse they experience, but it also helps them envision an alternative, speculative future in which our reproductive decisions are socially and economically supported and enabled.

Reproductive Justice helped reinvigorate another movement now called birth justice, to which this anthology is a long-awaited addition. In the words of Molly Arthur, one of the contributors of this anthology, "Anyone who believes that the right to be born into health and love in a just and flourishing world should be supported and protected is a BirthKeeper." I guess that makes me a BirthKeeper, too, because I believe in birth justice.

This anthology is a welcome and vital contribution from the voices of healing and compassion of those choosing to help others through the birthing process. The writers reimagine the birthing process in a non-capitalist fashion, highlighting the interdependence of humanity that is challenged by the "medical industrial complex" that robs people of agency, self-determination, and human rights. BirthKeepers broaden the ability of people to take charge of their own reproductive journeys. Starting with childbirth education as a radical practice, the birth justice movement has forever changed how we view our bodies and our rights to control our reproductive decisions.

I wish every young person received quality childbirth education from BirthKeepers as a human right before such knowledge is urgently needed in the delivery room. The contributors to this anthology are making that new world of birth justice possible and inevitable. I am honored to be in your presence. Thank you.

Preface
Victoria Law

When my daughter was born in 2000, both activists and most media saw parenting and politics as entirely different realms. But over the past fifteen years, tales from the parenting trenches have become more accepted in the political discourse, from mothers of color reflecting on raising biracial children to parents of murdered children leading local fights against police violence.[1] These stories show what some of us have been saying all along—parenting is not only personal, it's political and is an integral part of a political community.

But where are the stories of the birth workers, midwives, doulas, and herbalists? Where is the recognition that their roles go beyond the limited time periods of pregnancy and birth that they redefine what we think of when we think of reproductive labor and care? After all, care is not just the process of supporting, birthing, or parenting a small child but also encompasses the mundane tasks necessary for daily survival, such as cooking, cleaning, and providing emotional support and sexual intimacy. These voices and experiences show us what Alana Apfel accurately calls "the immense potential for personal and systemic transformation inherent in this work." But, since these tasks are rarely considered waged work, they continue to be overlooked in discussions around labor.

Birth Work as Care Work positions this type of work at the intersections of labor and Reproductive Justice. Coined by women of color in the 1990s, the term "Reproductive Justice" covers the full scope of women's reproductive lives, including decisions about whether and when to have children and the ability to raise these children with dignity. But unlike the traditional reproductive rights advocates, those fighting for Reproductive Justice also recognize that the decision to have— or not have—children is also caught up in societal inequities. As Asian Communities for Reproductive Justice explained, "Reproductive Justice exists when all people have the social, political and economic power and resources to make healthy decisions about our gender, bodies, sexuality and families for ourselves and our communities. Reproductive Justice aims to transform power inequities and create long-term systemic change, and therefore relies on the leadership of communities most impacted by reproductive oppression."[2]

"But I'm not planning to have kids," you may protest. "Why should I care about Reproductive Justice? And why should I read this book?" Reproductive care and labor illustrate the power inequalities inherent throughout the United States. Reproductive justice stands at the crossroads of race, gender, sexuality, citizenship, and class. Social justice organizers need not be planning to start families of their own to recognize the power dynamics inherent in how social injustice impacts self-determination.

For instance, whose work is worthy of compensation? Whose work is marginalized and expected to be performed for free? In "Labors of Birth Work," Apfel describes the undervaluing of care work in which people (usually women and particularly women of color) are paid to care for the children of other families. In the meantime, they are expected to leave their own family responsibilities.

In the 1970s, second-wave feminists such as Selma James issued a demand of Wages for Housework, positing that the unpaid work that women were doing in the home—from caring for their children and other loved ones to cooking, cleaning, grocery shopping, and all of the other tasks that keep a household functioning—should be recognized and financially compensated.[3] While certain sectors of the women's movement took up the call, the broader Left did not, and the following decade, with the election of Ronald Reagan in the United States, the idea that women should receive any money for staying home to care for their children was not only disparaged but vilified. In the United States, welfare mothers were demonized as cheats and drains on society. Women's gains began to be measured in terms of their ability to climb the corporate and political ladders in capitalist America while the realities facing their less white, less monied, less resourced counterparts were dismissed. After all, as one white mother wrote in the 1990s, didn't everyone have a job that not only paid handsomely but also offered full benefits, including paid maternity leave, and onsite day care?

But these power dynamics are not limited to the "Lean In" crowd. The Birth Justice Project, a volunteer group, goes into the San Francisco County Jail to provide reproductive health education and doula support to women locked within. Apfel's interview with these doulas illustrates how race, gender, and class come together to block certain women's access to birth and Reproductive Justice. Even during birth (or birthing), social justice (or injustice) matters. In yet another interview, Jodi Koumouitzes-Douvia, a doula, domestic worker, mother, and public health graduate, points out, "All the structures that exist outside the hospital are felt inside the hospital and sometimes even more intensely."

Doula Sophia Perez echoes this observation, giving example after example of the institutional racism and class differences she's witnessed in medical care.

> You see the ways in which black birthing people are assumed to be high-risk and have certain illnesses, which may or may not be the case. People who do not speak "good" English are yelled at. Loud women are told to "keep it down." Alternative family configurations are

not often considered, let alone respected. Transgender birthing people are treated in a way that diminishes dignity and respect. There are assumptions about black fatherhood and motherhood. There is also a blaming for one's health. Patients covered by Medicaid are spoken to repeatedly about contraception, because they are perceived to be a burden. Unsolicited advice and assumptions about people's levels of knowledge are heavily informed by classism. People who are pushed into the margins, due to racial/economic/disability-based oppression are likely to be the same people whom most often have their needs and humanity overlooked.

For Perez, and for the other contributors, birth work is social justice work. Perez connects Reproductive Justice organizing to more well-known examples of social and racial justice organizing. For instance, how many scholars of black liberation are aware that the Black Panthers worked around reproductive health? Some still do—former Panther Erica Huggins trained the East Bay Birth Support Project, a collaboration between the Birth Justice Project and Black Women's Birthing Justice, both of which address health and access disparities by providing support for people of color birthing within low-income and underserved communities (including jails). As part of her training, Huggins included some of this little-known aspect of Panther history, drawing a connection to the Panthers' survival-pending-revolution programs in the black community and today's fights for Reproductive Justice.

This past year, I spent six months interviewing women about being pregnant while incarcerated throughout the United States.[4] Mothers often spoke about feeling isolated and helpless. The night before her scheduled caesarean section, for example, Kandyce was locked in a room in the prison's infirmary. There, she had nothing to take her mind off the impending birth—and the guaranteed separation from her newborn less than forty-eight hours later. "All you do is sit in this room by yourself. You know you're about to have your baby [and] that you're going to have to give your daughter up. All you have time to do is to think about it." What would have helped, she said, was to have a support person. "Just a voice to listen, somebody to talk to you about what's going on," she said.

Having a doula would not have remedied the insubstantial food, hours locked in a room, and the prison's unwillingness to address the needs that accompany pregnancy. But it would have provided that listening ear that Kandyce so needed—and the feeling that her experience and her care mattered. But the prison does not have a doula program and so she spent the night with only her thoughts and anxieties for company. The experience was so stressful that, even one year later, she told me, "I don't ever want to be pregnant again."

All of the interviews and essays in this volume combine practice and theory. Whether you ever plan to have children in your life, read this book and think about Reproductive Justice not just as an issue for individual parents and children but as an integral part of the larger struggle for justice and community.

Introduction

Silvia Federici

As Loretta Ross, cofounder of the SisterSong Collective, reminds us in the foreword to this work, the rise in the mid-1990s of a movement of African American women fighting for Reproductive Justice has transformed the politics of the field. By establishing the fundamental principle that as crucial as the right to refuse unwanted maternities is women's right to have children and to have them under the conditions they want, Reproductive Justice activists have broadened the struggle over reproduction, to include the demand for social justice, and in this process they have also begun to transform the conditions in which women give birth.

Alana Apfel's *Birth Work as Care Work* is a powerful contribution to this project and to the perspective of the birth and Reproductive Justice movement, which refuses to see women as victims and instead stresses their capacity for resistance and self-determination.

Constructed through interviews with doulas and midwives reflecting on their experiences and the objectives of their practice, the book is a perfect entry to understanding why *birth workers* have become an important presence in the birthing room, and why they see their activity as political activism and a key aspect of the broader struggle for human liberation.

Birth work, we learn, is more than advocacy work, needed to shield expectant mothers from a medical system steeped in misogyny and racism, or an alternative to the heavily managed, Taylorized delivery that hospitals provide. A central theme in all the interventions that compose the book, embodied in the image of the delivering woman as a warrior, is that birth work is above all a transformative, autonomy-building activity, enabling women to "take charge of their reproductive journey," overcome their fears, discover their inner powers, turn the moment in which they are most vulnerable into one in which they can be strongest and, thereby, begin a process of self-valorization.

This is a revolutionary project, whose significance transcends the experience of childbirth, as it expresses a view of political activism and social change that I believe is essential to every form of struggle. This is the view (central to my own work) that the construction of an alternative society must begin with a profound transformation of the activities by which we reproduce our lives and the relations that sustain them. For to the extent that capitalism attempts to appropriate every moment of our reproduction and to subordinate it to needs of the labor market, this is the terrain where we most often experience our first defeats. It is the terrain where we learn that our lives have little value, that we must curb our desires and practice self-discipline and self-denial, in preparation for a future whose course presumably will be decided by others than ourselves. To break with the constraints that capitalism places on our capacity to reproduce ourselves and our communities according to our own desires is therefore an essential condition for the construction of a society built on the principles of justice and self-determination. This is where birth work, as described by Alana Apfel and the other contributors to this volume, is paradigmatic of the ways in which we need to transform our reproduction, as the first act of refusal of the devaluation that proletarian women and especially women of color have historically suffered in their encounters with the institutions, and the first act of re-appropriation of what is undoubtedly one of the most important experiences in a woman's life.

It is no accident that this begins with the recreation of the community of women that in the past participated in this event, before it was placed under the control of the medical profession. Contrary to the ruling ideology, the advantages that medical innovation has produced have hardly compensated for the loss that the increasing exclusion of midwives and neighbors from the delivery room has implied. As in the case of many other activities, the breakdown of cooperation in the process of reproduction weakened women's resistance to the intervention of the state in their lives. Not only were midwives often most knowledgeable, owing to their broad experience, than the doctors who replaced them. Being assisted by other women, who often had a direct experience of childbirth, was a great source of strength for the expectant mothers, who could trust the goodwill motivating their efforts and benefit from a collective knowledge that women had transmitted through the generations.

It is one of the merits of *Birth Work as Care Work* that it demonstrates how the principle of the "commons" operates in the delivery room and, more specifically, how, even today, in moments of potential crisis, the presence of BirthKeepers is as important as any medical know-how for the success of child delivery, for this greatly depends on the value the participants place on the child to be born, and their ability to communicate to the mother the necessary trust in her own capacity to carry on the task.

There are other aspects of *Birth Work as Care Work* that make it a politically important document. The intensely poetic character of the writing in "Tales from the Birth Field," the section in which Apfel describes her work in the birth room, is riveting, as the prose evokes the rhythms of the birthing process and the excitement that accompanies the birth of the new child is communicated to the readers, driving us to think of our own birth, of our relation to our mothers, and of the profound connection between life-giving and dying.

Another reason for the power of *Birth Work as Care Work* is that it avoids the moralizing tone that at times permeates the language of the promoters of "natural birth." The book does not set a model of procreation to which it expects women to conform, aiming instead to awaken the consciousness in us of our innate abilities and powers and introduce us to a different kind of politics, in which the moment of resistance and confrontation is not separated from the reproduction of everyday life. It is a politics whose importance is only now beginning to be recognized by many social movements: one that demands that our struggle must at all points be constructive, not only opposing institutional violence but refashioning the social fabric of our communities, and prefiguring in its forms the world it wishes to build. It in this sense as well that Apfel speaks of birth work, and more generally care work, as already a "political activism," and the book itself—in its language and in the way in which it is constructed—is an example of this principle.

Alana Apfel has not only given us a theoretical analysis of birth work in its all different dimensions and birth-stories that exemplify them. She has also ensured that the reader has all the instruments necessary to fully understand and appreciate the book content and its political importance, introducing, for instance, a very helpful Political Dictionary that immediately gives us the backbone of the book and ensures that no one has to feel humiliated because they do not understand what the terminology that is used implies. The book also includes a chapter with useful information about herbs and plants that reminds us of the all-important connection between the care of the earth and the care of the body, and the necessary alliance between the Reproductive Justice movement and the environmental and ecological movements, as well as the movement against land privatization and enclosure.

Birth Work as Care Work will inspire its readers. I was deeply moved from the first few pages. It was perhaps reading

Loretta J. Ross's vivid account of her postpartum encounter with her child or Alana Apfel's recollection of the last words in her mother's journal. Whatever the cause, I knew right then that this would be a great book, one where the words are already an action, and repeated readings have only confirmed this judgment.

A BEGINNING

Birth Worker as Activist

We cannot build an alternative society and a strong self-reproducing movement unless we redefine in more cooperative ways our reproduction and put an end to the separation between the personal and the political, political activism and the reproduction of everyday life.

—Silvia Federici[5]

There is no such thing as a single-issue struggle because we do not lead single-issue lives.

—Audre Lorde[6]

This anthology gives voice to the activism of birth workers within radical reproductive struggles. You will read stories from the front lines of activist birth communities, hearing from birth workers, midwives, doulas, herbalists, and those who choose to align their labor with the production and reproduction of everyday life. Birth holds many possibilities for transformation and birth workers, as activist caregivers, frequently find themselves as key political mediators in this process.

The aim of the anthology is to provide a platform for activists to reflect on and articulate the political and social dynamics of birth work within the context of larger liberatory movements. The featured stories herein envision the reproductive process as a unique moment that enlivens, and indeed is grounded in, the very essence of social and political life. The anthology will appeal to all those interested in the dynamics of human struggle, reproductive labor, and birth. It speaks, in particular, to birth workers and activists in the hopes of strengthening birth and Reproductive Justice struggles and reminds caregivers of the immense potential for personal and systemic transformation inherent in this work. It also speaks to radical theorists and those with an interest in social movements with the intention of expanding recognition of care and care work as direct forms of political engagement.

What do we mean by "care work" in the context of birth? Care work has long been identified by feminists as an essential, yet highly undervalued, form of labor to capitalist society.[7] It may involve the provision of emotional and social support, sexual intimacy, companionship, and looking after children as well as more mundane daily tasks such as cooking, cleaning, shopping, and running a household. The majority of these activities take place within the imagined "privacy of the home," which has the effect of masking their true significance to the continuation of every social and economic system. Care work is by nature *reproductive*—it is the labor that ensures that the individual and community are properly sustained, nourished, and reproduced anew each day. It is a necessary precursor to all forms of capitalist (re)production. But within an environment that associates "real work" with labor that takes place *outside* of the home, the result is a degradation of the labor of caregiving communities whose struggles are contained and importantly *depoliticized* within the so-called private sphere. Yet the climate in which both reproduction and caregiving unfolds remains anything but "private." The terrain of reproduction continues to be highly contested and itself a site of resistance—for wherever capitalism exerts control over how we seek to reproduce ourselves and our communities, we find acts of rebellion, however small, that bring us closer to a collective re-appropriation of reproduction from capitalist patriarchy. *Where better to begin than with birth itself?*

Starting from this premise, and with a specific focus on the care that accompanies birth, the contributors to this anthology explore the political and *politicized* relations that run throughout all reproductive experiences including fertility, abortion, birth, miscarriage, and rape, as well as between birth work and other forms of social struggle such as prisoner rights, racial justice, or environmental activism. In so doing, they break down the distinctions between public/private and personal/political and embody the logic of what Silvia Federici calls a "self-reproducing movement."[8] This means that they do not view their "political work" as separate from the work they do in supporting the reproductive experiences of others and in reproducing the collective body as a whole—for what is a social movement if not a struggle over the texture and reproduction of life itself?

In collapsing the personal and political, the figure of the activist birth worker emerges shedding light on the book's central theme: to highlight the unique contribution of birth work within intersectional struggles for self-determination and justice and to draw attention to the politicized nature of caregiving under capitalism. Birth workers, particularly those who work independently, dramatize the intersection of the personal and political because they occupy a space that is at once inside and outside of medical authority. This is because while they work, most commonly, *within* hospitals, they work *for* themselves, enabling them to bring a certain degree of subversive freedom and institutional critique to their practice. From this position, as expert caregivers and mediators of reproduction, they can avoid being "medicalized," leaving them with the potential to confront and redress institutional forms of violence that are inflicted upon reproductive and birthing bodies. Fashioning the birth worker as activist in this way casts caregiving itself as a potentially radical form of activism that holds the ability to literally reimagine our life beginnings. Activist birth work here joins with other liberatory movements resonating beyond hospital walls to reinvigorate the commonalities of our human existence. As Molly Arthur states in this anthology, "We are all born through birthing bodies and we are all part of the physicality of this world." Birth and death are what bind us together.

In critically engaging medical institutions, activist birth work also sheds light on the complex systems of power and privilege that are often at play in the reproductive context. Institutionalized privilege goes hand in hand with institutionalized oppression leading some to benefit and others to be harmed. This gives rise to huge reproductive health disparities and a frequent silencing of the specific needs of a person in labor. In these situations, some or all of a person's intersectional identities may be disregarded, leaving medical staff with more authority in charge of the unfolding reproductive experience.

Here contributors draw on the teachings of Reproductive Justice in broadening the political discourse of childbirth reform.[9] They seek to demonstrate that all discussion of sexual and reproductive "rights" must also always address the intersectional context in which rights attached to people might be exercised. This means acknowledging the effects of historically oppressive structures and their role in shaping sexual and reproductive oppressions across time. Without enough emphasis placed on this analysis the result is a movement which predominately reflects and upholds the demands of economically privileged and female-bodied white women while overlooking the reproductive experiences and injustices of marginalized communities and communities of color within political organizing. This is not to underestimate the hard fought victories of feminists and reproductive health activists in gaining the level of reproductive freedoms enjoyed by some today. The changes that arose in the aftermath of the "scopolamine era"[10] and the radical political movements of the 1960 and '70s have had a profound effect on the revival of midwifery,

5

women's sexuality and health education, and the rights and well-being of birth givers the world over.[11] The intention here is to build on this history yet also to go deeper in understanding the effects of intersectional oppression on childbirth and following from this, to expand and diversify approaches to birth activism as a result. As Jeanne Flavin reminds us, the fight for *all* birth givers to be considered "fully human" rages on.[12]

With this in mind the anthology approaches birth and reproductive activism with historical awareness of the particularities of reproductive injustices and with the intent to confront narratives of birth that mask and perpetuate reproductive injustice. One such problematic narrative relates to the language of "choice" within modern maternity care. The danger of celebrating the rise of choice within transactional birthing environments lies in masking ongoing forms of coercion that result in a denial of choice for marginalized communities and those with less access to the kinds of choice-making power enjoyed by more privileged counterparts. This framework suggests that the individual retains full agency in decision-making over their health while overlooking, and therefore masking, intersections of race, gender, sexuality, physical ability, citizenship, and economics that differentially affect health outcomes and determine the quality and extent of care that is given. Health care in the United States is far from "choice-based"; it is deeply embedded within existing systems of social and racial stratification that produce highly variable birth outcomes across a diversity of reproductive communities.

In the United States, women of color experience the highest rates of cervical cancer, HIV/AIDS, sexually transmitted infections, diabetes, and unintended pregnancies, and regardless of socioeconomic background are more likely to die in childbirth than white women.[13] Here, we see that although the physical experience of pregnancy and birth may hold similarities across different communities, the systems of governance that shape and often determine how individual births unfold are clearly *not* the same. Economically disadvantaged communities, communities of color, and queer and gender-nonconforming communities in particular bear the brunt of institutional forms of violence. Sophia Perez, for example, demonstrates how systemic forms of oppression as well as health and economic disparities felt in the outside world are also present in the labor and delivery ward. This is particularly evident through the "managing" or pathologizing of black and brown bodies in the birthing process. Rather than being purely biological, individual birth outcomes emerge out of a myriad of racial, sociopolitical, and economic forces that are structurally produced and reproduced throughout time. These forces collide, often violently, in determining the sexual and reproductive trajectory of entire communities. Breaking cycles of oppression means directly engaging these systems in order to reimagine a language of birth that creates room for all birth givers to have supportive reproductive care. In so doing, activist birth work interrogates institutionalized oppressions and critiques profit-driven health care models while reinvigorating a conversation about body-autonomy and sexual and reproductive freedoms throughout society.

A central element of the activism represented in this anthology herein focuses on broadening the nature and language of care to incorporate a greater diversity of reproductive needs. Not everyone experiences their sexual and reproductive bodies in the same way and to subsume all birth givers within the same form of reproductive care is often to erase individual identities and lived experiences. Different histories require different forms of attention. Here a politics of social change is rooted in the *particularities* of lived oppressions while still maintaining affinity to a larger common struggle for human rights in birth. This leads to the emergence of differentiated forms of care as well as community-led birth and reproductive support that we see addressed in this anthology. The anthology also makes a conscious effort to break with definitions of care that are articulated within a "provider" framework. This is seen to reproduce relationships of inequality in which those who may have more knowledge in a particular field, like birth, are deemed legitimate in taking charge of other people's reproductive experience and thus of forcing onto others their own version of how bodies should or shouldn't behave. Birth workers hold space for others to discover their *own* inner potential, helping facilitate but never taking charge of the trials, joys, and beauty that come from navigating one's own reproductive journey.

In supporting birth givers to realize their own strength through birth, birth workers help destabilize the fear-based foundations upon which the modern labor and delivery ward is based. This not only serves as a challenge to and subversion of traditional spheres of "reproductive labor" (both literally and figuratively) but also undermines the very structures of capital that differentiate and ignore these spheres of work. As Silvia Federici notes in the introduction, the effect of capitalism is a continued appropriation of all aspects of our reproduction, which become subordinated and devalued to the needs of the profit-driven market. What this means in the reproductive context is not only control over how, where and with whom we give birth but also control at the level of *imagination*—foreclosing the ability for people to literally imagine alternatives to, say, lying flat on your back or having your baby separated from you at birth. We need a collective re-appropriation of the constraints capitalism places on our imagination around birth and hence on our capacity to reproduce ourselves and our children in ways that would support our collective well-being. In order to move closer to this we would necessarily need to enlist the direct participation of *all* caregiving communities—especially those who have been historically silenced. This would mean far more decision-making power granted to those whose bodies serve to sustain, reproduce, and literally give life to all others, yet who are also most often disenfranchised at the moment of reproduction. If we revitalize anti-capitalist modes of relating—weaving cooperation, liberatory politics, and respect for all beings together with the immense physiological capabilities and spiritual power of birth givers—we might have the beginnings of a truly revolutionary birth movement.

A Note on Organization

Birth is neither a linear nor predictable narrative. What follows is an attempt to capture a sense of this dynamic motion through an assemblage of intersecting thoughts, embodied experiences, remedies, and recipes that come together to weave a web of subversive change and attempt to tell a story of contemporary birth under late capitalism. Not all contributors agree with each other, nor are they encouraged to do so. The diversity of approaches within birth worker activism is honestly reflected. The intention of this collection is to turn relationships of perceived difference into politically productive partnerships capable of destabilizing dominant narratives of birth. In so doing, the anthology aims to elaborate new ways of thinking, acting, and relating, mediated and given shape through our reproductive experiences. The anthology opens with "Birth Story," a short tale of remembering that weaves birth work together with maternal lineage. "Organizational Practice" presents a recollected conversation with two activist birth workers exploring the essence and texture of social justice organizing within the context of birth and reproduction. "The Labors of Birth Work" makes up the majority of the text and presents a series of collaborative and co-created interviews that explore a diversity of perspectives and approaches within the field of birth and reproductive activism. All examine dynamic and creative ways to reimagine collective engagement with birth and reproduction centralizing birth work and birth workers as key political mediators in this struggle.

"Tales from the Birth Field" presents four birth stories, inspired from real life events and told from the perspective of a doula. The stories are included to paint a picture of birth work as it is experienced in the moment, with all the smells, physical feats, and transformation that both giving birth and supporting birth entails. The hope is to transport readers directly into the surreal, and often mystical, world of birthing, bringing context and real-life experiences to some of the more abstract themes addressed throughout the anthology. This is followed by "Herbs for Pregnancy, Birth, and Beyond," a practical resource of remedies specifically geared towards supporting pregnancy, birth, and postpartum. Readers are encouraged to think of these plants as their supporters, teachers, and friends during these transformative times. Herbs are included to highlight the importance of exploring alternatives to mainstream medications, emphasizing solidarity with our natural environment. Finally, the "Political Dictionary" is included as a way to unpack the political language and terminology of birth and reproductive activism with the intent of uncovering deeper meanings and significance. It is intended as a reference that can be used throughout the anthology.

An Experiment in Radical Well-being
This anthology identifies itself as part of the common intellect circulating tools for the achievement of radical well-being within a shared space for health and healing. Radical well-being means health and healing from the bottom up. It means birthing without fear; reclaiming and furthering our knowledge of herbal medicine; having proper support through all reproductive experiences and outcomes; elaborating radical love with each other; and working to collectively create communities of care, strength, and vitality that stand in opposition to capitalist modes of relating. It also means recognizing the connection between access to and knowledge of health and healing and global systems of circulating power. It means striving to bring

knowledge of health back to the commons and into the hands, hearts, and bodies of the majority, facilitating the coming to power of our fullest selves in the direction of healthy social change. In so doing it adopts what might be called a prefigurative approach to social change—embodying through one's actions the very world one wishes to bring forth. This means starting from the grassroots health of the community in order to create a loving and livable world in the here and now. Birth seems a pretty good place to start, don't you think?

Birth Work as Care Work is a de-centered, multivocal, and co-created narrative. Rather than a "complete" text, it casts itself as one offering among many directed towards the collective re-appropriation and celebration of one of life's most essential struggles. Let the text herein be an invitation for further dialogue, mutual learning, and collective action. The hope is to encourage readers to recognize the subversive potential inherent in birth work, care work, and all forms of labor that serve to produce and reproduce our collective society. The reader might productively carry on where this anthology leaves off—perhaps through sharing positive birth stories or pursuing further study in birth work or perhaps simply through reinvigorating their own numerous and unique daily acts of resistance, in whatever way this may be defined. Ultimately the anthology is conceived as a platform through which to honor birth—in all its forms—as itself a profoundly radical act that holds the potential for deep transformative change.

Birth Story

"You are the guardian of all I was and will be."
    —From my mother's last journal entry, 2003

The first moments of life outside the womb are some of our most sensitive, vulnerable, and memorable. They mark the beginning of individuated life experienced with deep and raw intensity. Our births may be remembered with enthusiasm or cut through with pain, yet each and every one tells a story of transformation, strength, and deep courage. Reconnecting with our own birth can function as a way to reconnect with the core of ourselves, a way to shed new light on the labor of those who give birth and to better understand the multiplicity of environments into which each person is born. Birth stories inspire, anger, make us weep, and call us to action. The following piece was written after a gathering in which we were asked to share the story of our birth and explore how this informs our practice as birth workers.

•

Explore any recurring images you have. Reflect on your approach and attitude to transitions and begin to reconstruct your own birth experience as you remember it best.

We are gathered on the floor of the living room to hear our speaker, a therapist who focuses on the importance of re-engaging our own birth story. The speaker asks us to form a circle, puts on some music, and passes around big pieces of paper and colorful pens. I choose a purple one.

I catch myself doodling on the side of the page. Small inter-connecting loops that slowly get bigger and bigger until they fill the whole page. This is a recurring behavior of mine. I try to focus back on her prompt. Everyone else seems to be writing furiously. My first thought is apprehensive confusion. Who can possibly remember their own birth? Yet, after sitting and thinking for a while, stories told to me by my parents start to resurface. These are mostly little anecdotes about who was there, the time of day, the atmosphere. All start to piece together an imaginary of what it might have been like. My page starts to fill. I begin to recite some facts. Born 2:22 pm, September 18, 1989. How heavy? Don't know. How long? Again don't know. Looking around I see furrowed brows and more than a few blank pages. Perhaps everyone isn't finding it as easy as I thought.

The speaker encourages us to ask our mothers for more details about our own births. I feel my heart ache. I knew this would come up—in fact it's partly why I'm here—but I wasn't prepared for this immediate surge of grief. My mother died when I was thirteen, something I experienced as a deep and painful shattering of my life. I feel hot tears on my face. Maybe it's because I feel so passionate about birth and know it's the work she also did. Maybe it's because I know this kind of con-versation ultimately remains closed to me. I'm still searching for answers. I long to ask her what she was thinking, feeling, and experiencing as her body contracted and opened to bring me to life. I don't know any of the people here well but I don't feel embarrassed as I let my body feel its grief. The speaker reaches over to me. "What do you need?" she asks. She doesn't tell me "it's OK" or to "take a minute outside," she just lets me cry. Tenderly she guides me to the floor and asks Tanya to rest her hands on my back. "Birth is a kind of dying and dying a kind of birth. These transitions are in many ways the same."

I feel Tanya's hands on my back like a grounding weight. It feels very nourishing. *Dying is a kind of birth.* Discovering or perhaps *re*discovering birth has begun to function as a way for me to remember my mother. This in the sense of piecing together an imagined sense of what our adult relationship would or could have looked like. I have been reconstructing this relationship through gathering stories and retracing our collective steps. Earlier this year I even sat in the room where I was born. From here I dreamed of my birth.

I was born at home, in a room that held many stories of transition—stories of beginnings and endings, of birth and death. My brother was born in the same room as I was, and my grandmother passed in this room two weeks after my birth. I think my mother was incredibly tapped into the power and energy of these profound transitions. As a mother with a terminal illness and as a midwife, she taught me to honor and never to fear the great power inherent in birthing and dying bodies. These lessons continually infuse and guide my practice as a doula and birth activist and as a guardian of transitions in my own right. Our birth stories are, in a sense, never really finished. They expand and contract through time ever deepening our connection to our mothers and to those who produce and reproduce the world to give birth to us anew each day.

Organizational Practice
Giving birth to the world we want

This piece is drawn from a recollected conversation with two activist birth workers. It examines challenges of leadership and representation that can arise within grassroots political organizing and explores the value of consensus decision-making and collective leadership within activist collectives. The dialogue also discusses the need for greater self-reflection among birth workers particularly in situating themselves within a political climate that engages differential power dynamics (such as that which exists between a birth worker and a pregnant inmate). The featured birth workers are part of a volunteer organization that provides reproductive health education and doula support to those who are incarcerated or formerly incarcerated. In 2014, this organization was awarded an eighteen-month grant from the Department of Public Health intended to expand the work and presence of the collective in their local county jails. This grant was a huge source of pride, but it also caused difficulties within the group, particularly around issues of collective representation both privately and to the newly watching public eye. The challenges of social justice organizing and of working within the prison industrial complex run throughout this conversation.

•

D: The nature of our volunteer organization has always followed the attitude that if you want to get involved you can. Everyone has been welcome in one way or another. This has meant that we have had a vast diversity of women wanting to work with us. Some are new doulas and some seasoned. Some have come with a clear political agenda and others with an "I'm just a giving volunteer" kind of attitude. I think it's great that we have made a point of welcoming everyone but this has often meant that women have turned up with very little idea of what it actually means to work within the prison industrial complex. The grant has meant a lot and has opened up new opportunities for growth and development but it has also triggered internal rifts that I don't think we were really prepared to deal with. I think a lot of these women could have done with examining some of their own privileges and cultivating a more critical awareness of their position within the jails. These things are important to think about, and as an organization we haven't always been as direct as we should have been in voicing these realities and examining ways to beneficially engage with these complicated dynamics.

Another question has also been whether we want to formulate a clear and fixed definition of who we are or what we stand for *before* bringing people in. Can we let that structure emerge naturally from our practice? Is our collective the people within it or is it something abstracted that people *secondarily* fit into? If we made the whole thing more formal how would this affect the cohesion of the group or our sense of collective identity and ability to make decisions together? Are there times when we need representatives to speak on behalf of the group? Does everything have to be consensus? These are all questions that are becoming increasingly relevant as we gain more attention and are particularly pressing if we choose to go down the NGO route for more funding. There have been times when I have acted on behalf of the group and should have communicated more with everyone. It's so hard to coordinate everyone's schedules. We are all volunteers, have other jobs, studying, or on call for expectant mothers so it's difficult to bring everyone together. I don't want to be part of the NGO-complex of always chasing money but I want to get things done and I think this is a real chance to use this money to expand much further.

A: It's a difficult task to maneuver between an identity as a radical organization on one hand and on the other as a group that accepts money from big governmental funders. Of course this will change the dynamics of the group. The more you operate from within structures set by governmental bodies or funders, the more limitations you experience. Do you explicitly present formal structures of identity in hopes of attracting more funding or do you remain a more fluid collective evolving from the shifting dynamics of the group and the specific work you are doing? Can theory or more coherent structure come from practice itself? I can see your worries of "selling out" and becoming another "NGO moderate" but maybe there is a way to walk a middle path and play the system to your advantage. This would mean finding your point of entry through entering into a formal relationship with governmental institutions (the route to public funding) yet once "in" acting with more radical intentions than are first apparent, kind of like a subversion of the very structures that work to constrain you.

D: This is what we have been developing in the jail. When we first arrived we were always under the watch of the guards. They sat in on every class. Now they have gotten to know us a bit. We've been coming for about two years now, so they've settled down. This has meant we have been able to greatly expand the sort of things we talk about. There are times when things get really sexy in there! We discuss some pretty radical sex education. Other times we can be very political. We have much more freedom now but this has come through dedication and time and to a large extent through initially adhering to the authority of the jails—at least to a point where they trust us.

17

E: At the same time our project isn't just an attempt to make the experience of jail more "cushy" for women but one of radical transformation. I'm a prison abolitionist! Not everyone in our collective is, though, and that has often been part of the problem. We don't all share the same political direction.

A: It is important to theorize where your personal politics fit into a broader project of social or political transformation. It might be useful to reflect upon the ways in which your beliefs about incarcerated people, discrimination, the prison indus-trial complex, or simply the role of doulas in underserved communities affects your approach to birth work as well as what you ultimately wish to see come of your collectives work. As you say, it's more than simply making the jails more "cushy" for women. What is this "more"? Do you for example intend to directly engage with the state through the medium of your collective? Is direct engagement always necessary to effect change within prisons and jails? Are there other ways of approaching this from *within* the prisons themselves? What does the political project of your collective actually look like? Or what *could* it look like?

D: My aim has never been to simply improve the relative comfort of women within jails (though this is vitally impor-tant) but rather to fundamentally transform—perhaps even abolish—the system of prisons entirely. Birthing in an envi-ronment of continuous support without violence or trauma. Who knows the true extent and effect this might have for both mother and baby? Deepening women's knowledge of reproduc-tive health is a crucial means of empowerment and strength that has significant effects beyond the confines of the jail walls. I am working to dismantle racism, homophobia, sexism, and class discrimination among a group of women who are disproportionately affected. This is not just about reform-ing prisons or jails but about radicalizing and empowering a group of women caught within a system that works to repeat-edly oppress and criminalize them.

LABORS OF BIRTH WORK

The Co-created Interview

The following stories are the result of a collaborative and co-created interview process. The interviews initially began with a series of framing questions used to situate the contributors politically and socially in relation to larger liberatory movements. Contributors were encouraged to explore their own understanding of "activism" within the context of birth work and to reflect on who the "we" might be among the loosely organized collective of birth workers that call themselves activists. Who is included and who is left out of this "we"? What implications does this have for the unfolding of care (both given and received) and the elaboration of different forms of reproductive activism? Is there a need for differentiated forms of care? What might an ethics of conscious birth work look like—where, when, and how to intervene and when to let be?

The contributors address these questions in diverse ways. Some call for an end to "white volunteerism" and the need for more people of color led birthing initiatives, others critique the dominance of heteronormative language within childbirth movements. Still others warn of the dangers of an unrealistic and elevated discourse of "natural birth" which works to shame those who cannot participate while also overlooking the power of hospital structures in determining the contours of reproductive experience. All highlight the unique role of birth workers as activists and political mediators, within a diversity of intersectional liberatory movements.

The written text gathered from the interviews went through several rounds of co-editing until all contributors felt content with the representation of their words. The interviews were an exercise in multivocality and co-creation that resulted in rich and dynamic final pieces. The final texts have been edited to remove the interview questions themselves in order to centralize the voices and stories of the contributors. Their work shines through as exemplary of the potent and transformative convergence of the personal and political in birth work, care work, and all forms of reproductive struggle.

Jodi Koumouitzes-Douvia is a full spectrum doula, domestic worker, mother, and public health graduate with a focus in maternal health. Jodi is also co-organizer of the Santa Cruz Doula Salon, a monthly community-based educational gathering of doulas. Our interview focuses on Jodi's experience as a doula, domestic worker, and public health graduate exploring ways in which these intersect to inform and shape her role as a paid caregiver. Jodi raises concerns about the undervaluing and invisibility of care work as both a mother and a birth worker. The interview concludes by addressing the need for differentiated forms of care to meet a diversity of needs that arise among different reproductive communities.

The field of public health is built around the concept of "interventions" to promote health. As a graduate student specializing in maternal health I started thinking about doula work in these terms and realized that the act of supporting someone else in labor *is* an effective form of intervention. This became the basis for my thesis, which presented research on doula care as a form of health intervention capable of producing beneficial outcomes that could support the whole family. Through this research I wanted to identify the effects and methods of doula support. I wanted to understand the reasons why women who labored with the support of a doula tended to report more positive birth outcomes and were significantly less likely to have an epidural, caesarean section, or episiotomy. What I found was that doulas were supporting mothers and their partners in a very tailored and unique way. One of the things about being a doula is that you have the opportunity to get to know your clients and be there for them for whatever they may need. Every woman is different and every birth experience is different. We have a lot of leeway to customize as doulas, and there are many different ways of giving support. One thing I've come to appreciate is that it's kind of a lot to ask partners to be there 100 percent. Some people just don't like blood, shit, or vomit. It's not everybody's scene. This may be their first time with a laboring woman. As doulas we are trained in birth, and are in many ways somewhat obsessed with birth. We really get to know our clients and become an integral part of whole the birthing experience.

The Undervaluing of Care Work

As a doula, it's always shocking to me that I get paid to take care of other people's children but not my own. People like Christine Morton, who published *Birth Ambassadors*, talk about the undervaluing of care work in this way. One helpful quote of hers I often think about says: "The caregiving dimensions of doula practice, a predominantly female occupation, can be compared with the contradictions and tensions emerging in other types of care work, paid and unpaid."[14]

I have done a lot of nanny work and childcare and have even combined this with my doula work. Right now, for example, I have a homebirth client with a toddler. They told me they needed someone to help clean and do childcare, so I told them I would do everything, childcare now and doula work later. This way I can form a relationship with their first child. I'm glad because now when I arrive to do my doula work this little boy will know who I am. I won't be a stranger in his house while his mother is having a baby. So I'm getting paid to be a part of their household but I'm not getting paid to take care of my own child.

We have to think about the social and political responsibility of doulas as part of a global community of care workers. This is something I struggle with because I feel like, on one hand, it's my social responsibility to take care of other women because we can and should support each other. But I also recognize that I never get paid to take care of my own family and because of this I get less time with them. Then there is the decision to give your doula services away for free because the belief is that this is a social and political movement and this is what you should do. The relationship between doulas and money is a complex discussion because I also feel like it's my social responsibility to charge, and to charge what I'm worth. This work deserves to be valued. The whole topic of responsibility in doula work and balancing one's personal passions and beliefs with other social responsibilities is difficult. Another quote of Morton's that helps me situate all this mentions: "It is especially important to examine how the emotional component of intense caregiving work can be seen not merely as an example of economic exploitation and gendered essentialism, but also as a motivating factor for the work in its own right."[15]

One of the biggest challenges as a doula, for me, has been navigating the intensity of power dynamics in the hospital. They are like an invisible force underlying everything and significantly affect the type of care that is possible. Physicians, nurses, lab techs, custodians, and patients—this is a very stratified group of people in the room all at once. The outside world constantly collides with doula work. All the structures that exist outside the hospital are felt inside the hospital and sometimes with even more intensity. Through my public health background, for example, I am very aware of the disparity in health and pregnancy outcomes for women of color. Even when you take away economic status, women of color still have the worst outcomes.

The majority of doulas that I know are white and straight, and the reality is that these folks probably aren't the best people to offer support to communities outside of their own. What we are seeing now, especially in places like the Bay Area, is something similar to the critique against second-wave feminism, which was led mainly by white, middle-class straight women. Many amazing birth workers of color are saying to white doulas, "We have something different to say!" I think this is great and totally needed. We need to challenge and move away from a discourse of white women "saving" people of color. White birth workers need to find respectful and appropriate ways to support from a far. This conversation is uncomfortable for many white folks but is absolutely essential. What I took away from the conference organized by *SQUAT*, a radical midwifery journal, was a call to support already existing projects rather than coming into communities and attempting to impose new agendas or start unwanted projects. Communities of color, especially birth workers, are absolutely capable of creating necessary forms of care and support from within. Recently I was introduced to the concept of "cultural humility" as an alternative to "cultural competence." It is extremely unrealistic to think we can actually become "competent" in all cultures. "Cultural humility" on the other hand encourages people to be honest, humble, and respectful about where other people are coming from without claiming to know everything about their reality.

One of the great things about the doulas in Santa Cruz is that everyone is willing to share their wisdom, experience, and training with each other. When some of our members go to conferences that others can't afford they bring back the notes and give us all the training. When anarchist friends of mine tell me they want to train to be a doula but don't have the funds I say: forget the training, come to our meetings and apprentice with somebody instead. Why not go outside of the usual norm for doula trainings? I'm not saying these formal institutions are worthless. Doulas of North America (DONA) has been a great jumping-off point, but again it comes from a white privileged background.

There is no official licensing agency or state board for doula work, and this means a lot of creative leeway. Yet sometimes this makes me feel powerless, and that's why I want more training particularly around abortion doula support. Abortion is so politically charged. The dynamic of public/private and personal/political is embodied in abortion all at once. Rights are being taken away and even access to birth control is being threatened. Taking action for me begins with not being silent.

I am proud to call myself a full spectrum doula. I see this work as very closely tied to feminist activism. This is feminism. This is about women and their bodies. It's about having choice and access. It's also about finding ways to support things that are going on in our own communities. It's also about listening and respectfully acknowledging when to let other communities do things for themselves. All of this is really hard when you work under a for-profit health care system and when you live in a capitalist system and need to feed yourself and look after your family. It's very hard to always volunteer your services. It's hard to be a full-time activist. There is no easy solution but there are a lot of small things we can do. It's about opening up the dialogue and getting new conversations started.

Kelly Gray is an educator, storyteller, collector, and activist. She worked as a union organizer for public-sector health care workers, was one of the founding members of the Bay Area Doula Project, and sat on the board of *SQUAT*, the radical midwifery and birth publication. Kelly now works at a small birth center in California and has begun training to become a death midwife. She wrote a column for *SQUAT*, The Other Side of the Coin, featuring stories of marginalized people and experiences in an attempt to have more conversations about the affects of cultural narratives on reproductive experiences. Our interview explores Kelly's efforts to reconfigure the language of storytelling to create new platforms for Reproductive Justice that make space for all to have supportive and appropriate reproductive care.

As a union rep I organized resident-physicians in community hospitals in both urban and rural settings. My job description was pretty basic: handle grievances, challenge the boss, negotiate the contract, and mobilize the workforce. What I found was that this work was actually that of a storyteller. As a union organizer, it's on you to create a culture that values the ongoing saga of public hospitals and the workers within them, both the history and the vision. If you are lucky, you are called upon to tell these stories in times of vulnerability. When a career is at stake, when a hospital is threatening to close down, when everyone knows that medical mistake can be avoided if a specific policy were changed or when a boss is humiliating a worker. This is when union members listen because this is when they are vulnerable. You are able to reach people and offer them a path to challenge and transform the status quo, but only if they are uncomfortable with the status quo. Otherwise, you're just that union rep who brings the pizza to meetings. And if you can't tell a compelling story, you'd better have brought good pizza.

This kind of storytelling is not so different from that of the birth worker. As a birth worker you provide a historical context and a vision so that people can walk a path that serves their needs, be it physical, cultural, spiritual, or emotional. Often I find that I support women in challenging predominant cultural narratives about how they should or should not experience their reproductive bodies, whether it's birth, pregnancy, infant loss, abortion, rape, or menstruation. These narratives have been passed on from generation to generation, taking root in our brains and in our DNA. We begin to see them as inevitable in our own unfolding life. As we internalize these stories, that childbirth must be painful or scary, or that we must remain silent around rape or miscarriage, we become profoundly fearful of forms of oppression created within our own minds and bodies. We hold on to unresolved grief and this lingers in our bones, our relationships, and our very being. This builds cumulatively from one biological experience to the next, creating chronic stress. Then we drag it all into labor. When we are stressed, we create the hormone adrenaline. This adrenaline, biologically intended for the last moments of birth, acts to shut down all of our systems during labor, including the production of the hormones that facilitate childbirth. These hormones—oxytocin, prolactin, endorphins—act as a link, or portal, to the profound and surreal worlds of birth, orgasm, and death, bringing us closer to the trancelike state of love. My job as a storyteller and educator is to tell a deeper and more ancient story where it is safe to sit with these sensations of being vulnerable because that it how we become powerful.

I learned as a union organizer that if you don't have a vulnerable workforce, you can't expect to see change. You must reach a certain level of agitation and suffering—the dark before the light—prior to transformation. We are collectively experiencing this darkness in the culture of hospital birth today, as reflected in the World Health Organization's recent declaration to stop abuse and disrespect in facility-based childbirth.[16] These injustices disproportionally affect people of color, queer and trans folk, and poor families. The level of violence, oppression, and misinformation that is common-place in hospital birth has led me to form very specific views about my personal role within that process.

When I started as a doula, my intention was to help families have empowering births, but in truth I found that my work was more about helping people process the abuse and disre-spect that they encountered in the hospital. Or, worse, some didn't even notice how horrifically they were being treated because I was so effective as a doula. I began to see myself as a part of the problem because I believed that as a society we would need to hit rock bottom before we start the transforma-tion, and I was acting as a bandage. Now, although I appreciate many doulas and the work that they do, I can no longer prac-tice as a doula for low-risk clients who choose a hospital birth because I can't allow myself to profit from an experience that takes place in an institution based in patriarchy and capital-ism. I cannot encourage people to have low-risk births within a system that frequently denies them their choices, dignity, and body autonomy. I have done work with high-risk pregnan-cies in hospitals and found this work profoundly life-altering and satisfying. Through my own journey, however, I have dis-covered that I am more interested in facilitating a conversa-tion around the link between sexuality, birth, death, loss, and reproductive experience and how we have the opportunity to transform each of these experiences. I have found that my work is radical when I focus my efforts on childbirth educa-tion because I can plant the seeds of an entirely different yet ancient story. The authoritarian medical model is very uncom-fortable for me and thus has become the basis of my activism as a union organizer, doula, and childbirth educator.

I find that the cornerstone of my work is to reconfigure the language that we use in our storytelling. One example is the misuse of language by people advocating for "natural birth." They paint a picture of flowering vaginas and perfect moms with painted bellies, "ohm-ing" their way through labor.

I think that in a typical hospital birth, where women and families succumb to the medical model of childbirth, it's absurd to expect a laboring person to have the tools and resources to obtain a natural birth. A laboring person will face everything from medical jargon that is attached to a slew of procedures and protocols, complicated power dynamics, group observation, and a hand reaching up her vagina while she's lying on her back with her legs open. Try going to poo with someone poking your rectum while your family watches—it's not going to be pretty. Under those circumstances, natural birth is reserved for those privileged enough to have escaped an abusive background and/or secured enough financial resources to hire a doula and attend a lengthy childbirth class.

When we anchor ourselves to the language around natural birth, the result is an industry that supports white woman privilege while silently shaming those who can't afford, emotionally or financially, to participate. By creating a debate between natural and medicated birth, it implies that the choice is solely that of the person giving birth, as opposed to the culture of the hospital and insurance companies receiving them. Our ability to ignore the realities that most people face while birthing in the hospital is self-defeating. If we can shift our language to reflect the desire to create avenues for all people to have supported births, no matter their socioeconomic backgrounds, race, gender, or personal history, then we are more likely to increase the percentage of people having natural births and reap the health benefits as a society. When I talk to my students I am careful not to give verbal value to natural birth over medicated birth, because I trust every person to make the choice that is right for them. However, I do emphasize the need to create a safe and supportive environment for every birthing family.

SQUAT: A Radical Midwifery and Birth Publication

SQUAT invited the participation of folks who are actively working to redefine birth justice. In my column, The Other

BIRTH WORK AS CARE WORK

Side of the Coin, I have interviewed folks who are working in full spectrum care and are involved in feminist, race, and gender struggles. We talk about how this work—often seemingly unrelated to birth work—actually has a deep effect on birth workers. For instance, issue 18 of *SQUAT* featured an interview I did with a woman who generously shared her grandmother's story of rape and how this story has shaped her work as an anti-imperialist feminist. The prior issue featured an interview that I did with one of the grandmothers of death midwifery. We talked about the commodification of death and the creation of the funeral industry. The funeral industry's history uncannily mirrors the move towards facility-based birth and the commodification of maternity care. I always attempt to bring it back to birth work in hopes that our readership can feel supported in creating commonalities between these experiences; rape, colonization of communities, commodification of biological experiences, traditional death and birth rituals. At *SQUAT*, it has been our hope to foster and feed a community of birth workers who can use any one of these stories as a lens to examine different approaches to birth work.

Many of my clients start a conversation with me by asking, "What if they force me to do something that I don't want to do with my body?" or "When will they take my baby away from me?" These questions are significant because they show us how our culture interfaces with the medical establishment. People see their doctors as authorities with complete control over their bodies and their babies—to the extent that they *expect* to be raped. The word *rape* might sound extreme, but I am quick to point out that when someone does something to your genitals without your consent, that is rape. For many families, this is the expectation about what will take place in the hospital, though they don't often use the same language as I do. We have to talk about informed consent and the importance of it, not from a legal perspective, although that's important, but from the equally important notion that when we invite people to touch us, we must give consent to keep our dignity intact. When two adults consent to intimate intercourse, it's lovemaking. When one adult does not consent, that's rape. You can see how your view of this one experience of intercourse both physically and emotionally hinges on consent. This is true of hospital procedures as well.

The families that I work with are not asking these questions as paranoid individuals, they are asking these questions because they are raised to believe that their life preferences and identities are insignificant and that their own bodies are shameful or scary. When you break down a community's ability to care for itself you open the door to oppression. From a very young age we are robbed of experiencing our biological functions as powerful initiations. Our sense of self begins to deteriorate. This affects how we experience menstruation and fertility, gender identity, sexuality, giving birth, menopause, and finally death. We have been force-fed commoditized versions of these experiences. We have let go of what it means to be human. Yet the human experience of life and death and all that is in between are the forces that bind us within cohesive communities. Working and creating art, growing food, eating, taking care of the sick, caring for the young and old, educating our children, birthing, supporting new families and the grieving—these are the functions of community. There are moments during and after birth, weddings, graduations, and funerals when you feel your compassion and desire to love and protect your community rise up inside you. You're flushed with oxytocin, which is the hormone that allows you to bond with those around you—you feel *connection*. A good rally will do the same—the music, the movement, the common vision. It's so seductive—it's an oxytocin high! Birth is a pause in life where you can momentarily break the silence of oppression and create connection. We are biologically designed to connect with others we just have to carve out space to do so. Birth, like abortion and death, allows us to hold up a mirror and ask the important questions: Who is making your choices? Who are you connected to? What do you value?

Laili Falatoonzadeh is a doula, activist, and member of the Birth Justice Project: a collective of doulas that provide reproductive support to inmates in the Bay Area jails. Our interview focuses on Laili's work with the Birth Justice Project reflecting on how power and privilege inform reproductive caregiving with inmates. The interview also explores the complexities of choosing where and how to practice midwifery in the United States, engaging questions of accessibility, institutional regulation, and liberatory struggles within birth and reproductive care.

The Birth Justice Project (BJP) was started by a group of doulas involved with the San Francisco General Hospital doula program. Several of these doulas learned from the doctor at San Francisco County Jail that incarcerated people deliver without any form of support other than the medical team at the hospital. Laboring people are checked by nurses around every thirty minutes, but apart from that they labor alone with guards outside the door. These doulas decided to form BJP so they could enter the jail system and provide prenatal and birth support to incarcerated people. Later on, however, it became apparent that as a group of primarily white doulas they were actually not the best people to be supporting communities of color and communities in jail because they didn't have the appropriate lived experience. So the direction of the organization changed, which included forming the East Bay Community Support Birth Project with Black Women Birthing Justice to create a training program for people of color and previously incarcerated people to become doulas. BJP was awarded a grant that provided funds for this training. The idea was that these people would have careers as doulas and be paired with a mentor that they would shadow for five births as part of their certification. We are continuing to work on the training as our first round of doulas move into the mentorship phase.

I am one of two doulas that currently provide support at San Francisco County Jail. There is an extensive clearance process that prevents more doulas engaging with this work. Access is very challenging, but those of us with clearance continue to provide regular prenatal and postpartum support to pregnant people. This typically involves a great deal of emotional support. Inmates receive a weekly checkup from nurse practitioners in Jail Health Services, but it's a pretty minimal amount of attention because the nurses are overwhelmed with patients. Nutrition is a huge problem. It is often at the discretion of the deputies to decide if a pregnant person gets an extra sandwich or not. We worked with a mom with gestational diabetes, for example, and the company that supplies food to the jail was never able to provide her with an appropriate diet, even after great persistence by the nurse practitioner over a five-month period. Maternal stress is also very high. A lot of my support work is really just telling people that they are a good parent and that they are strong. We also offer continuing services if inmates are released before their delivery date and we commit to being at their birth.

I'm really excited about the work of BJP. We recently had a retreat where we hunkered down into our vision and a lot of what came up was the idea of shifting the paradigm of "white volunteerism" into community supported systems—not just for birth work, but for everything! This means every community having access to resources and appropriate forms of support from within their *own* communities. Personally it's challenging for me because I am half Iranian and half white, but in the United States I am just considered a white woman. I'm trying to figure out what my role is here because I do want to support communities of color and allow people without resources to have access to the services I can provide. But I also don't want to be just another white provider. I'm really exploring what this looks like as a "white" woman through my work with BJP and my transition to midwifery.

Midwifery Today

There are a lot of different ways to approach becoming a midwife in the United States. It has been difficult to figure out where to place myself and I've been oscillating between becoming a certified professional midwife (CPM) and a certified nurse midwife (CNM). As a CPM I would go to an independent midwifery school and do a large amount of apprenticeship with elders while in school. This would set me up to do homebirths. As a CNM I would become a certified nurse and go to nursing school where I would specialize in women's health care and midwifery. This is a more medically orientated model where the majority of my training would be in the hospital. It's tricky because different states have different laws about where these different types of midwives can and cannot work.

The activist in me wants to become a certified professional midwife. I think this is the most radical type of work—the apprenticeship model. But it also has certain limits on the populations you can support. Not being able to be compensated through insurance and having folks pay out of pocket means many CPMs currently serve predominantly upperclass white women, which is not the only population I want to serve. Maybe there will be a shift towards greater accessibility. I think that in the future it's possible that CPMs will create a model that will be more able to cater to people of color and pregnant people without resources.

We haven't created a supportive environment for pregnant people to access midwives in the United States. There is a lot of fear being created around homebirths. Hospitals are touted as the safest place to have your baby, with the best technology. A lot of pregnant people feel uncomfortable about the idea of giving birth at home. I think there is a lot of miseducation out there. If there were more working homebirth midwives then people would be more accustomed to them as part of the birthing conversation. Policy is also very limiting. It's hard to be a practitioner in a culture where you

are liable for everything. Change has to start from a multifac-
eted and ground-up approach. On the other hand there are
also pregnant people who may not want to have a homebirth
because they don't have a home or they don't have a safe space
to give birth outside the hospital. It can be a privilege to have
a homebirth.

We are dealing with a patriarchy in our society that closes
down pregnant people's ability to express themselves. There is
a lot of oppression and repression that happens around birth
in our culture, but if pregnant people are able to access their
inner strength and trust in themselves and in their bodies,
birth can be transformative. They know they are capable,
deserving, and powerful, and this can translate into the rest of
their lives. One connection I made in my work as a community
organizer is that people who give birth are both nurturers of
the community and of the earth. If we have a disempowered
body of birth givers then we threaten the very fabric of our
society. Strengthening this could save all of our lives.

Cynthea Denise is a registered nurse, prenatal yoga teacher, postpartum doula and childbirth educator. Her nursing career encompasses all areas of maternal-infant health, including labor and delivery, postpartum, newborn nursery and NICU (neonatal intensive care unit). She worked in public hospitals for twenty years before choosing to start her own business as a prenatal yoga teacher. Our interview focuses on Cynthea's experience of working in public hospitals and explores the tensions of hospital hierarchies and power differentials that exist between doctors, patients and other medical staff. Cynthea also highlights the prevalence of racial and socioeconomic prejudice in the hospital examining ways in which these systems act to inform and shape how birth is experienced within the medical model.

When I worked in labor and delivery as a nurse, I would watch women give birth every day. There was often a lot of joy in the room but something never felt quite right about the way the process unfolded. It felt like a surreal experience because I would operate as part of the hospital and go through the motions but underneath I was constantly having doubts. I would watch women struggling on their backs or be subjected to all sorts of interventions and augmentations that would completely consume and direct their experience. I often felt really in tune with these women but someone else would come in the room and have a different perception and because of their superior authority would completely take charge of the situation. They did not allow these women to have their own experience. There were times when emergency caesarean sections were necessary of course, like when a baby had prolonged decelerations, but often nothing severe was happening and there was no indication for surgery. This really bothered me because I felt like medical staff just came in and made all the decisions on behalf of the laboring mother.

Most of these women would never ask *why*; they just went along with it. This made me realize the extent and power of internalized cultural norms. We have been schooled to believe that doctors have absolute authority over our bodies, always have the right answers and would never do us harm. This runs very deep. When I think about ways to "unlearn" this belief, I see it as beginning with women owning their bodies. Women can come to a place of greater autonomy in the hospital through a willingness to take ownership over their bodies and through finding their voice and sharing their stories. Yet this is difficult to achieve because there is such a pronounced loss of power when you come into a hospital. Even if you feel like you've got it all together, you come to realize that there is a deeply ingrained psychological component that is inclined to defer to authority because the hospital is experienced through relations of domination and a hierarchy of perceived competence.

This is a mentality I also had to unlearn. When I first started working as a nurse in an inner-city hospital, for example, there was a night when I spoke to a mother harshly because she had brought her child with her and was using the emergency room as a place to spend the night. I made some remark to her about the inappropriateness of using the ER as a clinic. My co-worker called me out after the shift. She pointed out that I did not know anything about this woman's situation and had made an assumption based on my own perceived notion of the appropriateness of her visit to the ER. My colleague taught me to accept every patient for who they are and to leave my judgments at the door. This really changed how I approached nursing. Later, when I worked at a hospital in East Oakland, there were times when I took care of babies whose mothers were out in the parking lot shooting up. I never felt like I had to "save" these women. They were adults making their own choices, and it sucked that they were using but I met them exactly where they were. I did not judge them. I listened to them and cared for them and their babies in whatever way I could while they were in the hospital. I felt at the time the best I could do was meet them in that moment.

One of the problems with social change movements whether focused on birth or any other issue is the mentality of being a "provider" for the less fortunate. Though the intentions may be good, what ends up happening is a reproduction of the idea that people with more knowledge or experience are somehow legitimated in taking charge of everything. This results in the dismissing of traditional cultures, opinions, or ways of life by those who seek to speak for others and implement their own version of "justice." There has to be much greater dialogue and understanding before people implement change or tell others how things should or should not be. The birth movement I am involved with is open and brings people together for these deeper dialogues. I think it is a movement of inquiry and respect that invites people to gather, share information, and listen deeply to each other. Transformation happens when we come together and meet each other where we actually are, not where others perceive us to be.

Prenatal Yoga
Through my practice as a prenatal yoga teacher I invite women to get into their bodies. There are many narratives circulating in our heads that take us out of our bodies, but yoga and meditation allow women to be more fully present in their bodies and to feel the connection between themselves and their baby. Practicing yoga offers the opportunity to shift perceptions about the ability of one's body to give birth. I really just give my students reinforcement about what is already happening in their bodies—a message that tells them their bodies are designed for birth and that they are capable and strong. There are many ways to experience birth that are different from what we have been made to believe. One student of mine, for example, recently realized she did not have to lie on her back to give birth. I told her that she could choose to stand, walk, squat, or kneel. This is a woman was operating with a prior belief system that made her to think she *had* to lie down and

that she had no power to question this narrative. My role as a teacher is to dispel old beliefs like this and invite in something new, enabling women to realize their own autonomy. Yoga is the vehicle through which I can be this catalyst.

I don't present myself as an activist. I prefer the word *catalyst*. This means I intentionally choose not to show up as an opposing force. I don't feel like presenting myself as opposing anything is going to be effective but I feel like catalyzing does. When you put baking soda and vinegar together, one is a catalyst for the other, and this *creates* something new. I'm more interested in being a creator and a catalyzing agent with deep intention. As such, I don't see the hospital as my enemy; I simply do not care to work or participate there anymore. I have come to realize I have a choice. For example, I have chosen not to participate in procedures like holding a baby down while a doctor cuts off the foreskin. By choosing not to participate in sustaining practices like this, I hope to show others that there is always a choice and always other options. We don't have to believe in the dominant stories told to us about birth. We can consciously withdraw participation from these narratives and create new stories, stories that have the potential to change the course of people's lives in a way that ushers in more peace and harmony on earth.

Yania Escobar is a full spectrum doula and community health activist. She has led membership trainings for the Bay Area Doula Project educating on issues of gender, privilege, and cultural appropriation. Our interview explores Yania's hesitation is becoming a doula and the unequal power dynamics that develop within caregiving. The interview also explores the dynamics of patient choice and what she perceives as a culture of shaming in relation to medical interventions during childbirth. Yania concludes by arguing for the necessity of full spectrum reproductive care and the importance of creating a more inclusive all-gendered birth movement.

The Bay Area Doula Project (BADP) is completely up-front about the fact that gender and race are central themes in our approach to birth work. Through our full spectrum doula training, we ask participants to reflect on what they really think and feel about these issues so that they can address their own baggage before they support somebody else. We have an exercise called "values clarification" in which people have to agree or disagree with certain statements and then discuss them afterwards. These statements may be something like, "People who use abortion as their main method of contraception are abusing the system." Participants in the training come up with all sorts of answers and the topics are highly debated at every session. Some people change their minds during the course of the training and others hold fast to what they believe. It's a very revealing collective exercise.

The biggest topic in our training program is abortion. Our focus is on having the right information: how, where, and when people can get an abortion as well as the costs and barriers to access. In my experience, as an abortion doula, I see a need for people to have much more information about abortion and to know their rights and options. BADP volunteers aim to demystify abortion and the different choices people make.

BADP is also concerned with applying radical gender identity awareness and practicing good standards of communication around these issues. We always say "pregnant person" not "pregnant woman," for example, because not everybody that is pregnant is a woman. It doesn't take longer to say "person" and it can make huge difference to inclusivity.

I consider myself to be a radical full spectrum doula. There is no other way I could envision offering my work. I want to provide support for any outcome—birth, abortion, miscarriage, stillbirth, or adoption—whether these outcomes are arrived at by choice, chance, or circumstance. I could never focus only on one aspect of a person's reproductive experience, that wouldn't feel complete.

One of the strangest dynamics among birth workers is that even though the majority of doulas work with pregnant people, most are actually childless themselves. I think this has to do with curiosity. I have to be honest with myself: I am curious about birth. I think it's something I'm going to experience one day and I'm curious about it. It's a major rite of passage. There is nothing wrong with wanting to witness somebody's huge life experience, but I think a large part of the draw for many doulas is to see what birth is actually like, in addition to offering support. This is similar to the rubbernecking that happens at the scene of an accident. Everybody says they are there to help but I think a lot of people just want to watch the birth and advance their careers. As a doula I'm scared that I would be a person who really just stares into the vagina to see the baby come out. As such I left my doula training very unsure about whether I could even be a doula, especially in the volunteer context. I don't want to take advantage of somebody else's poverty or financial situation for my own benefit. For example, I'm not OK with saying I'm going to translate for somebody and then expect this to give me full legitimacy to be part of their reproductive experience.

In addition, all of my birth training centralized on a discourse of "natural birth." The language used was always about "women" having a "choice" to feel the pain. That's all well and good but in today's medical world they also have a choice *not* the feel the pain and this should also be considered as a valid choice. If there are medical interventions available people should feel completely legitimized in having them. If somebody wants to get an epidural then they want to get an epidural! I feel like a lot of the training as a doula focuses on talking people out of getting epidurals, using labor-augmenting drugs, or getting a caesarean section. It is important to remember that just because people have more choices today, it doesn't mean we have to erase previous options. For example, just because some people want to squat, kneel, or stand doesn't mean that others don't want to lie down on a bed. All the choices are available to us. We don't have to move away from something in order to move into something else. There should be no limit to the reproductive choices we can have.

Intersectionality

Conversations about reproductive choice experienced as part of a radical gender analysis are already happening in other social movement contexts. People are realizing that you can't talk about gender if you don't talk about reproduction, so a deeper conversation about birth is becoming integral to these movements. In particular there has been a critical deconstruction of what the "biological" roles of people are or what our reproductive experiences are "meant" to look like. This sort of dialogue can be really difficult because, in the medical world, a female makes the egg and a male makes the sperm, and that's final. But it's also equally important to acknowledge that many people who self-identify as women have been fighting for a long time to be recognized and respected *as women*. I think the feminist movement has contributed a lot to reproductive rights and will continue to do so. Many in the birth movement know their struggles are interrelated in some way but they can't quite articulate how. As we get closer to the core of who we are as people—women, men, transgender, queer, or gender fluid—we get closer to the core of our common struggle. This in essence is the idea that everybody wants to be treated fairly and taken seriously. The birth movement is a fundamental part of this. My vision for a radical birth movement would be one that is truly all-gender-inclusive. Imagine what it would be like for babies to be born and for nobody to have to talk about their gender until the person whose gender is in question wants to. This means that, on an individual level, gender is not really an issue. The medical world certainly has a role to play in this transformation, but I don't want to depend on them to lead the change. In order to infiltrate society we have to work on media portrayals and everyday social interactions and normalize an engagement with gender fluidity in all aspects of our lives, not least with birth and reproductive experience.

ALANA APFEL

Molly Arthur is an environmental and birth activist and BirthKeeper. She is the convener of Ecobirth: Women for Earth and Birth, an organization that supports women who want to consciously change our culture's story to compassion for the environments of Earth and Birth and to impel social change to sustain healthy, caring humans and a healed earth home. Our interview explores Molly's desire to protect the "MotherBaby MotherEarth" bond; she urges a reclaiming of our maternal lines in order to explore the physical, ecological, and spiritual connections between earth and our right place in the world. She draws links between the destruction and excavation of the body of MotherEarth and the violence inflicted upon pregnant bodies today. The interview also examines intergenerational effects of toxic exposure on the physical and spiritual body of parent and child. The interview concludes by contemplating the future of both environmental and Reproductive Justice activism.

When my grandmother gave birth to my mother in San Francisco in 1912, she was probably given scopolamine, which was a commonly used drug in the early 1900s. Scopolamine is what they now call a "date rape drug"—ingesting it makes you forget. Women were literally made to forget their birthing experience, yet even though they were cognitively unconscious, their physical bodies still experienced pain. This meant that women often fought back and thrashed around, resulting in being tied down while giving birth. Medical staff would use lamb's wool for their wrists and legs because they didn't want their husbands to see the bruises that came from being tied to gurneys. What does it mean it be born into a terror like that or for a woman's body to go through that terror? In her conscious narrative brain the woman may not remember, but her body certainly remembers, her nervous system remembers. In the United States, we are born with the imprint of this legacy. Generations of people have this imprint. What are the implications for our society? How has this imprint inhibited our potential to be fully realized human beings? Where is the healing necessary for ourselves, our children and our future generations? My sense is that we need to look at our maternal line to understand the great importance of the relationship between MotherBaby and MotherEarth in order to reclaim our rightful place in the order of the world.

It is important for us to rise up in reverence to our maternal connectivity and to understand that the perceived differences that we have with all life are just that: perceived. We are actually, biologically, related to everyone. Our bodies are made of the cells of our ancestors and their environments. This can be traced through our maternal lineage right back to the very first starburst of life! So what do we do with this realization? We try and live in relationship and try to honor and support the bond that we have between people and with our MotherEarth. A great way to look at this is through the birth act itself. I am involved with a collective of BirthKeepers working to support and raise awareness about the relationship between MotherBaby and MotherEarth. Anyone who believes that the right to be born into health and love in a just and flourishing world should be supported and protected is a BirthKeeper. There is an evolved way in which we give birth as humans and a central part of this is the physical bonding we do during birth through the release of oxytocin, which enables us to love and to feed our children. Scientists have actually found traces of our children's DNA in our brains, blood, and throughout our entire body, years after their gestation. No wonder we have such a deep connection to our children! The interplay of the psychological and emotional with the biological is a fascinating endeavor to look at. BirthKeepers as a movement looks at the transformative potentials for us personally, for our world and for the future generations inherent in protecting the MotherBaby MotherEarth relationship.

MotherBaby MotherEarth

What we've been doing to MotherEarth is comparable to what we do to the human body. The mining and excavation of the bones and blood of MotherEarth is comparable to the altering and interventions done to our bodies. This needs to be seen and understood. For example, when a baby is born it can have as many as 250 pollutants in its cord blood. Our breastfeeding is now passing on poisons; our bodies become perpetrators of harm, even through the loving act of birthing and breastfeeding. This is very intimate and it is wrong. We life-givers have to speak up!

I look at the MotherBaby MotherEarth archetype and think about what it would look like if we put this first in our consideration? What change would we see in our society? The truth is the systems today are life threatening and life dismissing and therefore need to be changed. This is where I see the connections between environmental activism and birth. We are all birthed through a body and we all have a mother. If the fierce love commitment of the mother were broadened to look at all children and all life and to incorporate a relationship with MotherEarth, we would improve all our lives, our world, and the future for our children and grandchildren. But the drive of capitalism to commoditize resources that are of the commons and to monetize and privatize them in order to make a profit is contrary to any life-giving systems. Capitalism and birth become intrinsically connected because the effects of capitalist relations are physically embodied within us. In our current economic system, for example, there is no concern for the vast quantity of polluting substances that go into our bodies, and hence our babies, as a direct result of capitalist transactions. The main concern is about making profit and increasing the bottom line rather than the care and long-term health of MotherBaby. The unique profit motive and hierarchy of capitalism also seeks to control women's bodies because it wants to control their knowledge, intuitive capabilities, and reproduction. Women are the producers of the next labor force and are therefore essential to sustaining capitalism. The autonomy that women have is a direct threat to the current economic system. What might it look like if we considered our bodies and birthing itself as part of the commons, under a similar threat to MotherEarth's commons? This could spark a deeply felt understanding of the need for large scale, systemic change. I think this must come from the ground up, from grassroots resistance movements. This is the only way we are going to get anything done because the current system seeks only to maintain its hegemony. We need to unite and collaborate with all social justice and environmental health movements and recognize that it is only through dialogue and forming relationships across communities that real change can be realized.

I think the major challenge as a movement of birth and social justice activists is to figure out how to function as we want the world to be. How do we work together with people from diverse backgrounds and perspectives? How do we look at the systems from which we have come and from which we have benefitted and see the endemic inequities that have privileged some and oppressed others and still be able to co-create a better world together? BirthKeepers is committed to the functioning of a society that would put a non-hierarchical and maternal focus to the forefront of everything we do. It is the creation of a movement that actively promotes the force of nurturing love, where all voices of life-givers are heard, particularly those that are most affected by society's harmful systems. This goes back to a foundational need to invest time in truly and deeply understanding each other in order to get along, to build committed connections, using the beautiful relationship model of MotherBaby MotherEarth. The declaration of interdependence for a grassroots birth movement hereby stems from the immutable fact that we are all related. We are all a part of the physicality of this world. We are all born through birthing bodies. A strong and supported bond between MotherBaby

MotherEarth will enable us to make conscious and clear decisions about our lives and do the necessary actions for social change together. It will help us to look unflinchingly at the truth of the real harm perpetrated on us and by us, and on our precious home, MotherEarth. We have to integrate the grief of that realization and no longer consent to the harm being done. And with our authentic understanding of our right place in the world, within our lineage to our ancestors and our primal elements ancestors, speak up and act as the truly compassionate, loving, and caring life-givers we all are. We will become Beloved Ancestors to the future generations.

Jewel Buchanan-Boone is a doula with the San Francisco General Hospital. Her philosophy and approach to birth work are rooted in her passion for reproductive and social justice. Our interview explores the dynamics of working as a volunteer in public hospitals and in providing support to people who might not otherwise have access to care. The interview also addresses the need to break cycles of oppression within communities of color particularly in relation to generational trauma and stigmas that surround black motherhood. Jewel concludes by urging greater recognition of the embodied power of love that stems from birthing suggesting that this force could radically transform society if incorporated into other aspects of social life.

In American culture, birth has been demonized and overly medicalized. There is a popular assumption, for example, that all women who give birth must go through painful, horrifying experiences. To some extent this can be true *if* you don't have a good support system. This is why programs such as the San Francisco General Hospital (SFGH) Doula Program are so valuable, because they offer access to forms of support people might not otherwise have. Many of the women who give birth at the General come from very turbulent situations, so having someone there to support and love them through this vulnerable and transformative experience can be extremely healing.

As a volunteer doula with the SFGH Doula Program I work as part of a birth team of medical staff. I always try to understand the context of what's going on so I can understand why or how decisions are made about a laboring mom's body. One thing that helped me in the beginning was to learn how to be receptive to different styles of work among the medical staff. Some nurses are more sensitive to patients and others have a more rigid style. Learning and understanding where these folks are coming from and being able to ask questions has been really valuable in allowing me to provide the best form of care to moms. I'm always willing to check in, help, and take direction. This not only means supporting the patients but also supporting the medical staff in order to avoid negative power dynamics coming into the room. Sometimes nurses do get a bit sensitive towards doulas because they feel like we don't know our place or are overly pushy. But at end of the day we have to realize that it doesn't matter how we *personally* feel about something because we are volunteering for the hospital, which is a privilege, and thus have to go by their policies. Being a good doula in the hospital means figuring out how to make this work, because challenging a nurse or mouthing off to a doctor isn't going to help the doula or the laboring mom. Our collective goal is to bring both mama and baby through safely, and this cannot be accomplished by holding firm to ego.

The Politics of Birth Work

As a woman of color, my heart has always been in communities of color and in understanding the many ramifications of oppression and different ways that the system institutionally tries to eradicate black and brown people. This can be anything from sterilizing mothers (at times, without their knowledge or consent) or attempting to force contraceptive methods on women in low-income communities and in communities of color. This creates environments and relationships that are not healthy for our children to grow up in. There is a real stigma around black motherhood and especially around single motherhood. My work is definitely political in that I do everything it takes to help bring healthy, non-traumatized children of color into this world. I want to do my best to ensure that mothers, especially mothers of color, don't have to experience trauma in their birthing experiences, when we know this can be prevented or lessened through competent and loving care. Working against oppression begins with having healthy, well-rounded communities. I believe a lot of the trauma is held within our spirits. This is passed down to our children, who then repeat a cycle of trauma and end up being subject to more layers of oppression. Through my work I try to break this cycle and spread a spirit of love, compassion, and self-determination—trusting that you know what is right for your body and your children and that you can affect real change in your community. For me, this is activism on a spiritual level. Not all radical change must be synonymous with militancy, but I do think it is militant to love your people fearlessly and freely, and to fight for that.

Becoming a doula feels like the bravest choice I've ever made. It has given me the courage to do internal healing and has enabled me to push my own boundaries and start looking for my place in the broader context of life. I have found my calling as a doula and birth worker and have really come to understand the need for this type of work especially in poor communities and communities of color. To be clear, this perspective doesn't come from wanting to "save" folks in these communities, but from the desire to create safe spaces to express, create, and to birth. I also want to work in middle-class spaces. I feel that sometimes the more access you have, the less informed you can be, which also has an effect on birthing expectations and experiences. For example, there are more affluent moms in my workplace whose support of caesarean sections and medicalized birth is incredibly strong. They are set in a medicalized, privileged mindset and want to have what I call "births of glamour"—essentially painless, minimal effect to their bodies, and the ability to be scheduled—all with the intention of lessoning the "inconvenience" of the natural process of birthing.

I would like to work with these women and let them know that natural birth isn't something to be afraid of and that it's not just for "lower-class" women who can't afford the luxury of designer births. That said, I would like to point out the current trend in the resurgence of "empowering natural childbirth" has been relegated (in terms of visibility) to the ranks

of affluent white women who can afford the care of midwives, doulas, and birth photographers. While women at this end of the spectrum enable me to support myself from this work, it is definitely important to me that 25 percent of my practice is totally free. This is important to me because all women deserve amazing birthing experiences, regardless of life station, and because we can never be "too good" professionally to help people in whatever financial situation they are in. Being a doula means meeting women where they are at, on either end of the spectrum, and supporting them in their decisions on how they want to birth. That is the heart and soul of healing. We have to recognize that there are many incredible women out there without money who really need someone to love and hold them through this amazing process, *and* there are affluent women who need the exact same thing. I want to be part of this transformative healing.

If women were able to manifest the sheer amount of power it takes to birth children in rest of their lives, this society would stand on its head. It is a powerful thing when you have a lot of strong women handling things. To me, this looks like women across the board rising up against patriarchy through refusing medications and interventions that are not medically necessary. These interventions are usually implemented to control or expedite labor, hindering the natural birthing process as well as creating potentially traumatic experiences. I have seen women—especially in transition—tap into an infinite and profound power born directly from love and sheer strength of will. As a doula, no words can describe the feeling of taking a step back and watching a mother birth her child from that place. In our current state, patriarchy supports a fiercely competitive and inherently oppressive paradigm. Yet if we were able to collaborate with the kind of love and energy that is present in empowered birthing spaces, there would be no way all of the horrible things going on in the world would still be happening. To me, deconstructing patriarchy entails women trusting their bodies more and manifesting their inner potential to make this world something very different than what it is today. I believe that we are heading in the right direction and that our communities are benefiting and changing for the better.

Sophia Perez provides doula support and reproductive care to people of color and those who are LGBTQI, disabled, low-income, or incarcerated. She was trained through the East Bay Community Birth Support Project. This is a collaborative initiative that trains people of color and formerly incarcerated people to be doulas. This interview focuses on the ways in which this training has informed Sophia's efforts to address the ongoing health and economic disparities in communities of color. The interview examines the experience of being pregnant and giving birth as a person of color in the United States and demonstrates the potential for societal transformation inherent in elaborating more people of color–led birthing initiatives. Sophia recently graduated from Mills College in Oakland and will be relocating to the South to pursue midwifery.

I trained as a doula through the East Bay Community Birth Support Project, which is the collaborative project of the Birth Justice Project and Black Women Birthing Justice. Both of these organizations address health and access disparities and provide support for people of color birthing within low-income, underserved, and incarcerated communities. I believe this training program was revolutionary. It heavily honored the lived experience of every one of its participants. Our trainers were women of color, with the exception of two white women, who have fantastic herstories of social justice work. Erica Huggins, a former Black Panther, talked to us about meditation and the work the Panthers did with reproductive health and justice. Arisika Razak talked to us about the birth journey, where it begins, where it goes, and where it lands. She talked to us about body movement and encouraged us to move our bodies within the class, as a way of centering and recognizing the divinity of ourselves and others. Arisika acknowledged every single body including fat bodies, which was really transformative and healing for me.

We spoke of our own birth stories. We spoke of things we grew up understanding about birth. In discussing the ways in which our cultural traditions inform this work, we were able to identify similarities and further understand cultural differences, which promoted a deeper sense of cultural humility. I am fairly certain that these things are not being talked about in more mainstream doula workshops, such as DONA (Doulas of North America). The approach of our training was both holistic and medical. Our trainers felt that the more information we had, the better we could understand what can go on during childbirth, and this has proven very true for me. With the exception of one homebirth, the births I have attended have been in the hospital. After the training, I felt that I was able to effectively decode some of the medical jargon that is often thrown at birthing people. It is an added skill that can keep my clients more informed. I feel certain that this training gave birth to a revolution among all the trainees, but especially so for me because whenever a woman of color feels empowered, valued, and heard, that can only lead to greater revolutionary action.

Birth Work as Social (Justice) Work
Incorporating social justice into this work, for me, means making sure that the birthing people I support feel heard, have their wishes honored, and have access to the support they deserve no matter their economic resources. Birth is physiological, spiritual, transformative, and personal. It should absolutely not be at the whim of the larger medical industrial complex. I want to focus on healing and transformation as a framework for addressing trauma. A large portion of institutional racism is rooted in the medical industrial complex. The health and economic disparities, violence, and oppression in the outside world are also present in labor and delivery. In the modern hospital for example, you see the ways in which people of color are managed by medical professionals. You

see the ways in which black birthing people are assumed to be high-risk and have certain illnesses, which may or may not be the case. People who do not speak "good" English are yelled at. Loud women are told to "keep it down." Alternative family configurations are not often considered, let alone respected. Transgender birthing people are treated in a way that diminishes dignity and respect. There are assumptions about black fatherhood and motherhood. There are assumptions about non-native English speakers and their ability to understand what is going on. And there is also a blaming for one's health.

Patients covered by Medicaid are spoken to repeatedly about contraception, because they are perceived to be a burden. I once saw a lactation consultant tell a woman that the best thing about breastfeeding was that she wouldn't have to rely on social services to get the formula she would otherwise need, versus focusing on the actual health benefits to the parent and baby. The truth of the matter was that the parent had exclusively breastfed her other three children and knew the benefits firsthand. She did not need to be educated about the benefits. I wanted to tell the lactation consultant, "Black women breastfeed too, you know!" Unsolicited advice and assumptions about people's levels of knowledge are heavily informed by classism. People who are pushed into the margins, due to racial/economic/disability-based oppression are likely to be the same people whom most often have their needs and humanity overlooked. This is where activism and birth work intersect for me: addressing the needs and humanity of those who are pushed to the margins.

From Medical to Transformational

Hospitals are intense and scary. They are sterile, not just in cleanliness but in approach. Recently while driving to the hospital I said to one of my clients, who was having a high-risk pregnancy, "I know we have a visual birth plan but I want to ask you one more time before we park, how can I best support you?" And she told me, "Be my voice when I cannot be my own." I asked this of another client, right as she was getting ready to push. She replied, "Just be my sister. As if you were my sister." It is clear that birthing people who experience marginalization and oppression feel that they do not have a voice or support while giving birth. This is sad. One of the ways I try to shift the sterile and medical environment into a more warm and loving environment is through touch. I ask the birthing parent, before the birth, if they are OK with touch and me being physically close to them. Consent is such a big part of this work. When I am able to be physically active with my client during labor and delivery, medical staff tend to spend less time in the room. To be honest, I feel as though we make the work of medical staff easier when we are hands-on and physically active, though some medical staff clearly do not respect doula work. With that, I am very cognizant of not overstepping boundaries.

I am not a medical practitioner. A doula cannot be medicalized. I am a support, a cheerleader. I am there to soothe. I try my hardest to keep fear out of the room, as my doula trainer Linda Jones advised us to do. My job is to keep the birthing parent coping with their labor and delivery and keep them as far away from suffering as possible. And I do this through gentle reminders of support and that they have the final say in their birthing process (barring medical emergency). Birth is one of the few times people experience pain with a purpose, but frankly, I would like to see a shift in even calling it pain, though this doesn't mean I don't also honor people's experiences of pain.

How the "F" Word Informs Birth Work: Intersectional Feminism

All of the births I have supported have been those of people of color. I have been so humbled by the bravery my clients have shown in their birthing process. However, I am continually reminded of the ways in which medical staff work under preconceived ideas about people of color in the birthing process. This is not only confined to medicalized birth. Within the "natural childbirth movement" for example, which, as I understand it, was a movement largely led by white women, I have often seen the birthing practices of women of color and "third world" women used as some sort of ideal. There is this idea that women of color give birth in the field and keep on working. I can't dispute the truth in that but I can say that feminism has informed the natural childbirth movement, which in turn has had an impact on who becomes a birth worker. In fact much of what is seen as feminism today is still informed by white and middle-class women. In this framework, it is white women who get to decide what is best for all women, especially women of color. This does not mean that women of color have not contributed and informed feminist politics, because we have. Where would we be without Loretta Ross, Dr. Kimberlé Crenshaw, or Dolores Huerta? Yet the reality is when women of color do the same work as white women, we are not seen as "professionals." We are seen as doing our jobs, of being who we are naturally predisposed to be: maternal, caring, mama, mami, caregiver. This is not seen as our work, but simply what we *do*. One of my challenges is and will continue to be negotiating compensation for the work I do.

As a woman of color in a disproportionately white field of birth work, it is challenging, because "imposter syndrome" runs deep no matter how much value we believe we bring to the arena. I know I do good work and have received valuable training, but still I doubt my competence. I do find comfort, support, and inspiration in speaking with other members of my doula cohort. I am not the only one experiencing this feeling. In fact, many people of color experience this when they enter fields of work or education that is largely dominated by white people. It is just this constant nagging sense that I think too much of myself, and that I have inserted myself into somewhere I do not belong. Even though I do know I belong here, and that women of color are needed in this work. How I plan to change birth work is by showing up, again and again, and talking about our value and the value of our communities. The only way I know how to change things is to show up and make sure everyone is clear that I am not going anywhere. This is the same way we work against the health disparities within our communities. This work could very well bring better birth outcomes for poor people, people of color, and especially black birthing people.

The lack of confidence many birthing people experience stems from the hypermedicalization of childbirth and pain management. We are socialized to rely on medical practitioners to reduce our pain, more than we are socialized to believe that we have all we need, in many cases, to cope with the pain and discomfort of childbirth. As a nation, I feel as though we trust medical professionals more than we do ourselves, and that is scary. It is scary because we do not fully understand the intention and the consequences of a medically managed birth. I don't want to invalidate the pain and discomfort people experience in childbirth but I also don't want to discount the degree to which medicalized childbirth is a form of control. I would rather have agency, transformation, and confidence be the focus of an upcoming birth, much more than fear. Birth cannot be standardized any more than any other function of the body.

The idea that birth can actually be managed, which largely means the management of women's bodies, stems from patriarchal ideas that a woman's body needs to be kept subordinate. And when you introduce non-binary birthing people into this idea of bodies being managed, more intersections of oppression arise. One of my clients right now identifies as genderqueer, and they are a strong advocate for themselves. Being able to witness that self-advocacy and learn from them has been very powerful. I learn so much from my clients. Even within a birthing community that has the goal of working with marginalized communities the language used is still largely heteronormative, referring to everyone to as a "mama." I am constantly trying to reframe that for people in a way that makes sense. A large portion of queer vernacular is highly academic and not accessible to many people, so the message can easily be lost—for example, not everyone knows what "cis" means. Cisgender could be explained as a person who was born as a certain sex and their gender matches that sex. For instance, I was assigned female at birth, and I identify as a woman: I am cisgender.

I believe there is a political and social responsibility in being a birth worker. Sometimes I think I know what that looks like, other times I realize how little I know. I was determined to go into academia, but after attending the doula training, I am clear I want to become a direct-entry midwife. That excites me and it scares me, because I see the ways in which birth work done from a largely holistic and "natural" framework is not valued and can even be seen as dangerous. I do not want to be a nurse midwife. No slight to nurse midwives, but I have a difficult time differentiating how they are different from the delivering OB/GYN I experience in hospital. I understand the profession to be heavily medicalized, and that is not a narrative I want to participate in. I have a healthy respect for medicine. But I also have a healthy respect for the complete physiological birth process that does not, as a rule, necessitate medical intervention. Where do I see myself in this discourse? I am inclined to say I want to empower people, but people don't need *me* to be empowered. I want to witness and participate in a way that is appropriate and actually helpful and determined by the birthing people rather than me. I want to participate in bringing birth home, literally and figuratively.

TALES FROM THE
BIRTH FIELD

Anika *was born in a hospital in Northern California.*

I raise my hand to knock on the door, feeling my heart thumping hard inside my chest. I am walking into my first birth as a doula and I don't know what to expect. Inside I find Grace lying on the bed in her hospital gown. She smiles and gestures for me to come closer. I look around the room and smile at her husband Aru, who is sitting on the sofa surrounded by bags of chocolate chip cookies. "Grace's favorite," I'm told with a wink.

Grace is not actually "in labor" yet—she is here for an induction because she has gestational diabetes. She tells me she is waiting for the nurse to come in and administer Cervidil, a labor-inducing medication used to soften and "ripen" the cervix before labor really gets started. As if on cue, there's a loud rap at the door and the nurse comes striding in.

"All right, are you ready? When I place Cervidil, I put it in good. Right around the back of the baby's head." She stretches out the word "good," giving a forceful gesture with her hands. It all seems pretty serious. After a brief pause she holds up what looks like a tiny tampon then bends over and promptly inserts it into Grace's vagina. It seems quite uncomfortable to administer and Grace grimaces but remains silent. The nurse tells us that Cervidil is normally placed for a twelve-hour session. I glance at the clock. It is almost ten o'clock. The long game of waiting begins. I stay until Grace feels settled but then head home at around midnight. Inductions can take days, and I live close. Aru and Grace's mother spend the night awkwardly squashing themselves onto the couch in the corner of the room.

Nothing happens over the course of the night and in the morning a decision is made to start a second round of Cervidil. The day comes and goes with no change. I head home for the second time, making sure my phone is on loud and place it on the pillow next to my head. My bags are packed and I am ready to go at a moment's notice. I try and rest, mostly unsuccessfully. During the second evening the drugs take effect, and Grace reaches four centimeters dilation around nine o'clock. Then, a sudden flurry of text messages tell me her waters have broken!

I rush out the door. As I'm biking to the hospital, Grace calls me and says her whole body is shaking with intense pain. It's all happening at once. The nurses have given her Pitocin and the contractions are coming on strong. She gets an epidural while I'm biking over. When I arrive she is on the bed with fetal monitors strapped around her bulging belly and a blood pressure monitor on her arm. She smiles at me, looking exhausted. As I come close she pushes the bag of urine attached to the catheter under the covers, not wanting me to see.

Then among all the noise and frantic energy something begins to shift. You can sense a change in her body, her movements, and her sounds. She is turning inwards and beginning to connect with her child and the great task ahead. We stand beside the bed in silence and wait. Then the midwife comes in and checks her. "It's time," she says calmly.

All of our concentration goes to Grace. This is the moment we have all been waiting for. Nine months, and three days in the hospital, leading up to this moment. The midwife raises the back of the bed and we prop Grace up against some pillows. She is half sitting, half lying down as she grips her inner thighs, leaving white marks on her swollen skin. I lift one of her legs and the nurse lifts the other. The midwife tells us to count. I hesitate. I thought it wasn't good to count pushes. But I'm new

and overwhelmed so at the count of 1, 2, 3 . . . Grace pushes down
hard with each contraction. Veins bulging and sweat pouring.

The midwife puts her fingers into Grace's vagina and tells
her, "push my fingers out." Grace frowns as the midwife but
keeps her concentration.

There is no chatter anymore. Grace's eyes are closed. She
softly strokes her belly in between each push. Every part of her
appears attuned to her body and her baby.

"I'm talking to the baby," is the only thing she says.

Her eyes remain closed. The smell of the room shifts. Stale
clothes and the scent of hospital coffee are still there but something else too, something more. A sort of metallic smell. Blood.
We are getting closer.

"Keep your face nice and loose. If it's loose up there it loose
down here." The midwife grins and crouches on a stool posi-
tioned between Grace legs. Her hands are gloved and covered
with bloody fluids.

I'm still holding Grace's leg up in the air. Her skin feels
incredibly hot. I watch her closely and somehow her focus and
determined energy pass through me. I breathe with her, watching her belly swell and dip with each contraction. Her belly
button has darkened. A deep brown line leads the way towards
the vaginal opening. We all count together and slowly we begin
to see the head. A full head of black hair coming out between
her legs! I can hardly believe it. We are all surrounding her
now. Even her mother has risen from her prayers. Red rosary
beads left on the sofa. She is holding Grace's head whispering
words and gently stroking her hair. Things seem to be moving
with a different quality of time. I notice there is lipstick on her
mother's teeth. The air feels thick. The nurses are getting ready
for the delivery.

Aru moves up to take my position holding Grace's left leg.
The baby has passed beneath the pelvic bone. She is crowning.
The lower half of the bed is removed. A plastic bag lies at the
end of the bed to catch the "messy stuff."

"Once the head and shoulders are out I'll pass her over to you and you can catch the baby." The midwife looks at Aru. He is trembling. His eyes are huge black saucers.

Suddenly it's all happening. Three days of waiting but now it's all moving so fast. More and more of the head becomes visible stretching the vaginal opening beyond all imagining.

Grace moans and cries out, "Oh Lord. Oh Lord!"

We can see the face. Her tiny face! Then her shoulders! First one then the other then whoosh! Her whole body comes gushing out on a tide of blood and fluids and everyone is crying. Or maybe it's just me. Or Grace. The whole room is blurry through my eyes, and golden and vibrating. Oh my god. We are laughing and crying. Aru lays the baby across Grace's chest. Grace keeps repeating, "I love you," holding her baby. Oxytocin is filling the room. We are all ridiculously high.

This is one of the most incredible things I have ever seen. How did she fit through? Watch as she takes her first breath and wriggles her toes! She is using her lungs for the first time! The midwife clamps the cord. Aru picks up the scissors, trembling. Slowly he cuts the cord. "Baby is on her own now," the midwife announces to the room.

Eight minutes after Anika takes her first breath, the placenta is born. The midwife puts her hand into the amniotic sack and lifts it up so we can see the chamber where she lived and grew over the last nine months. It's absolutely incredible to imagine her in there. Flipping over the placenta you can see the intricate web of veins. They form a perfect tree of life. It's stunning to behold. Anika is wrapped up and a tiny hat is put on her perfect head of black hair. She is weighed and measured and brought back to Grace. After about an hour of nurses coming in and out and various tests being done it's back to just the family and the doula. The room is once again quiet and still.

"Would you like to hold the baby?" Grace asks.

My heart swells. I cradle her in my arms. She is so very tiny. I am holding a baby less than an hour old! This is truly the most vulnerable, intimate, and pure being I have ever been in the presence of. She looks straight at me with dark eyes and I wonder where she's been and what she knows. What did she experience, think, feel, remember as she traveled from the womb into this world? She takes great gulps of air and tries out her lungs with delicate little cries. Her eyes roll back in her head as she learns to focus and to truly see this world of which she is newly part. She opens her mouth looking for the nipple. How does she know to do this? What is learnt in the womb? My mind and heart are overflowing with wonder. True wonder at this tiny being who seems to know and recognize her mother's voice and her father's laugh. They have all taken this journey together walking in as pregnant woman and man and leaving as mother and father and daughter—as a family.

As we leave the midwife stops me in the hall.

"So you want to be a doula?" she says.

"*Yes!*"

"It's the greatest job in the world. The hours suck."

Lucy *was born at home in Northern California.*

Thaddeus texts me as 6:30 a.m.: *Joanna is having steady contractions. Can you be here in an hour?* I rise and start packing my bag having no idea how long I should prepare to be gone. If it's anything like my first hospital birth, it might be days. I arrive at 7:30 a.m. and Joanna is just getting out of the shower. She has been having regular contractions for a few hours but is still able to walk and talk coherently through them all. I help her alternate between getting on and off the couch and trying different positions as labor slowly intensifies and she works through each contraction. She seems to find the greatest relief by getting on all fours and cradling her head in her arms.

After a few hours her contractions progress into a regular rhythm. Walking seems to intensify things but this is becoming harder and harder to do as the time goes on. Conversation is slowing and demands are coming faster and sharper. It is time to call the midwife.

"Can I get in the tub yet?" Joanna pleads.

I am trying to delay the tub as long as possible. We don't want to blow all our tricks too soon.

"You meanie," she says. But she thanks me for it later.

Finally at around 3:00 p.m. we start filling the tub with hot water and Joanna slides in eagerly. Her pain immediately eases up but so do her contractions. Just as she is sinking into the tub Laurie, the midwife, arrives. I fill her in on the day's

ALANA APFEL

progression. I don't do vaginal examinations so I have no way of knowing how far along she is. Laurie checks her and pulls me aside to tell me she is three centimeters. Joanna asked not to be told. It's just as well—it doesn't help to fixate on numbers. She has a long way to go. Laurie sets up her stuff, settles in and then offers to collect the barbeque, Joanna's choice of post-birth food. Wrapping it in foil, she places it in the oven to keep warm.

Joanna is content in the birthing tub and takes most of her contractions with her legs spread and her back leaning over the edge. Between each one, her arms fly up behind her head and her hands open and close in silent communication. This is the signal that someone, usually Thaddeus, should hold both her hands as she works through the sensations. As this pattern progresses I notice that little things—a nail's scratchy edge or the sound of shoes on the wood floor—are starting to become more unbearable. In such an intimate setting every little sound or movement is intensified.

"Take off your shoes. Be still. Completely still," she says. The sound of the plastic liner rustling in the tub is causing offense. We didn't fit it properly and it keeps slipping down the edge risking getting the borrowed birthing tub dirty. Thaddeus tries to duct tape around the edges but the noise is too much and it's not sticking properly. He is getting really frustrated with this and keeps trying to pull it down between contractions. Joanna yells at him to stop. Laurie checks her in the tub. Still three centimeters. The baby's head is low and pushing on her rectum, causing a lot of the pain.

"I might go and come back," Laurie whispers to me.

"Water, water. Pressure!" screams Joanna.

I'm (not so) secretly hoping Laurie doesn't go. We all try and rest but every four minutes one of us jumps up to hold Joanna's hand through her contractions. This is full-on total attention work. We try to get her to eat some food but she keeps vomiting everything up. In the end bite-size pieces of banana with almond butter works best. She manages to eat a few bites.

I am on hot water patrol, ferrying buckets of hot water to and from the stove to the tub. Thaddeus is scooping cold water out. After a while Joanna asks me to stay with her and pour hot water over her back during the long, intense contractions.

I look up and notice it's dark outside. We've been at it for hours. Time moves so differently with birth. Then amidst the plastic crunching and the sound of running water I notice her sounds are beginning to change tone. There are still high-pitched screams but there is also something else, a lower, much deeper sound. My ears prick up. This is the sound we are looking for.

"Don't waste all your energy up here in your throat," says Laurie. "Try and send the energy down to your bottom."

Joanna lets out a deafening howl.

"That's you opening," say Laurie. "Try not to push. Blow air through your lips, it will help you to stop pushing before you're ready." She purses her lips and demonstrates blowing a raspberry.

"Water! Pressure! Water! Pressure!" yells Joanna. There are few other words. The rest of the room has gone silent, each person quietly and purposefully fulfilling their given role. Thaddeus rarely leaves her side, getting in and out of the tub as she needs and gently stroking her back when allowed.

"I'm not even close, am I? I feel like I'm ripping in half."

"You're doing beautifully. Baby is happy and healthy too."

Laurie places the monitor over her belly and we all listen to the baby's heartbeat. There seem to be very few rests between contractions. The howls are getting steadily louder.

"I can't do this. The baby is never going to come," says Joanna.

"Yes you can. You *are* doing it. Let me check you and see if you are ready to push."

Rebecca, the second midwife, arrives. She looks as if she has come straight from dancing—tight jeans, a black choker, and a flushed face. I remember that it's Saturday night. Rebecca is here to deal with the baby immediately after the birth. Her arrival seems to work as a good form of encouragement and motivation for Joanna. It means the midwives think she is close to delivery.

"You are fully dilated, Joanna," she says.

Fully dilated. The words she has been waiting for.

"How do I push?" she says, looking around wildly.

"Show her how to breathe." The midwives direct this at me.

Laurie is busy checking the baby's heartbeat. I think I can see a little of the head through the murky water but it's hard to tell in the darkness.

"All right, Joanna," I say with a confidence I'm not sure I have. "Trust yourself and follow your body. Let your body guide you. You will know when to push." Her breath slows and her focus deepens. She looks incredibly powerful.

Somehow she has made it through transition and pushing has begun. The long labor has paid off and now it's time to bring the baby into the world.

"Take off your shirt, Thaddeus. Take off your shirt," she says. Thaddeus looks at me and hesitates for just a moment. Then he rips his shirt off and jumps in the tub, cradling his arms around his wife.

There is a sudden sharp knock on the door.

I rush to the door and yank it open.

"What's going on? Are you OK?"

"She is giving birth."

"Birth?"

"Yes, *birth!*"

I slam the door shut and rush back to the tub. Is she crowning? There is definitely something happening. Rebecca listens to the baby's heartbeat.

"Everything is fine, but it's time to get baby out of the birth canal. Channel your pushes downwards. Sometimes making low, grunting moans with your pushes also helps bring the baby down. Try that if it feels right."

The baby's head is getting bigger and bigger. It feels somewhat surreal being with Joanna in this living room paddling pool, but the strength and focus she is exuding brings me back. She is at home giving birth to her child. I look around at the birth team. I can't see much under the water. Laurie's hands are under the surface and Thaddeus is right beside her. Rebecca prepares her equipment for the baby's arrival. Joanna is squatting in the tub and pushing with fierce determination. One more push and suddenly the baby's out! Thaddeus "catches" her and flops her on to Joanna's chest. She's incredible. She's done it!

Joanna seems, for want of a better word, startled by the turn of events. She is awestruck. I take my time to look around the room grinning madly at everyone. The room is hushed till Joanna laughs out in delight, breaking the silence.

"Are you OK with her not having a middle name, Thaddeus?"

"I'm fine, honey."

"What's her name?" We cry out.

"Lucy. It's Lucy," they say together.

The water in the tub is turning brown and cold to the touch. She has been in there for hours. We help her get up slowly. Blood runs down her legs as we walk her to the sofa. Rebecca throws a bunch of chuck pads underneath her. I have already covered the sofa with old blankets and towels. It's a patchwork of ripped beach towels and faded cotton. Baby Lucy looks so tiny. The midwives clean her up and cut her umbilical cord. We are still waiting for the placenta to be born. About ten minutes later it comes out with just a little pushing. I watch as Laurie holds the cord and helps guide out the placenta with only a small gush of blood. We all crowd closer with excitement.

Laurie lays the placenta out on a pad. It looks so beautiful and intricate, each vein forming the shape of the tree. "This is yours now," she says and flops the bloody organ right into my hands.

Lucy begins to cry softly. The midwives say she has the longest newborn nails they have ever seen. They are long and perfectly curved. One of her ears is a little floppy, like it might have been bent in the womb for a while. Her head is already re-forming into more of a head-like shape. She latches on and starts to feed. Joanna and Thaddeus cradle around her smiling. Love fills the room.

With a cheeky grin, the midwives take a little finger dab of "vernix," the white cream that newborn babies are coated with, and rub it gently around their eyes.

"Best anti-aging cream there is," they say, winking at me.

Madison was born in a hospital in Northern California.

I read a text from Donae: *I'm having contractions. Meet me at the hospital.* It's almost mid-February, maybe they'll get the Valentine's baby they wanted after all. At the hospital I find Donae's family already in the lobby.

"What's the news?"

"Donae is in triage. Only one person allowed in with her. Rafa has gone." They rest of us sit and wait. An hour passes. Then another. I turn my head at the sound of the elevator and see Donae walking out, looking exhausted but otherwise happy. Rafa, her partner, has his arm linked through hers.

"I'm not in labor. They are sending me home."

"Your body is getting ready in its own time," I say.

We gather our things and head home. The night passes with no calls and I manage to rest. Then in the afternoon I get another text. *I'm having steady contractions now. I think this is it.*

I head back to the hospital for day two and go up to triage with Donae. A nurse checks her and smiles saying: "You are four centimeters. We can admit you to your room now."

The room we get is reasonably sized with windows and a tub. It's always a lottery for the tubs! We begin decorating it with little trinkets from Donae's house. I hang bunting that spells out the word "love" over the bed. It's almost Valentine's after all. Some pictures and other keepsakes are placed on the table beside her. We are making the space our own, bringing a little of Donae's home and life into the hospital.

As the day progresses, Donae and I get into a good rhythm. When she feels a contraction I gently run my hands up her back as she breathes in and down her arms as she breathes out. One of the nurses, an ex-doula, gives me little battery-powered tea lights and we put them around the bath.

"I swear by dim lighting for labor," she says with a wink. I smile and thank her as I run the bath.

I hardly notice the time passing at first, but then, pausing to stretch my back, I look up and realize the daylight has faded. We are well into the night. My body suddenly feels extremely tired. I realize I haven't had a rest or sat down for well over twelve hours. A few more hours in the strain begins to take its toll. I can feel my eyelids burning from lack of sleep. Every limb aches. I look at the clock. We've been laboring for close to twenty-four hours now. Where did the time go? I haven't been out of the hospital in what feels like days. What *is* days. I look at Donae and her face shows determination but also deep exhaustion.

A new nurse comes in and asks if she can check Donae. We work hard to find a comfortable position for her to be checked but lying down is very hard now. Finally the nurse goes ahead but Donae howls with pain.

"Oh, that's right. I keep forgetting you don't have an epidural. I'm sorry. Looks like you're fully dilated though" says the nurse.

It's been over thirty hours of hard labor. Donae can barely stand up. She seems completely out of it as more nurses stride in and flip on the lights, announcing, "It's time to push."

The nurses set a bar across the bed. We try and get Donae into a position where she can pull herself up as she pushes, but the length of time she has been laboring has completely worn her out and she can't muster the strength to push effectively. We can even see the baby's head but the force behind the pushes is not budging the baby. I look around at the room.

My eyes are going blurry from tiredness but I see the nurses exchange looks with each other. I can sense that "caesarean" is on their minds. Donae's energy is clearly fading. We discuss options with the nurses and decide to get an epidural hoping this will allow a little rest.

Once the epidural gets placed, its effects are immediate. Donae falls asleep instantly. I take this time to sit down and eat something. I'm absolutely starving. A much needed rest for everyone. But just as I'm drifting off, the nurses come back in.

"We want to get this baby out now," they say. They point at the paper measuring the baby's heart tones and show me several prolonged declarations. These are points at which the baby's heart rate has gone down. They wake Donae up with a shake. It's only been about half an hour. Her contractions seem to have tapered off since the epidural. They tell her she needs Pitocin to get this baby out now. Their tone is urgent, probably for good reason, but it brings panic to the room. I try to remain calm and centered to support Donae. The Pitocin works fast and the contractions come back with force. We gather around her for her second round of pushes. Her husband is by her side speaking words of encouragement. I cradle my arms underneath her back, helping her curl upwards for each push. There is a mirror in front of the bed so she can see her baby, but nothing seems to be moving.

One of the nurses pulls me aside, the one who used to be a doula, and whispers, "I think we should try a vacuum extraction."

I haven't been part of as assisted delivery like this before and I ask her to explain more. She says a vacuum extraction is sort of like a suction cup that they attach around the baby's head. When the person giving birth feels the urge to push, the doctor uses the suction to help bring the baby down and out. It doesn't actually "suck" the baby out of the body but works alongside the person giving birth supporting a dynamic of push and pull to assist delivery.

"We wont have the option to use the vacuum much longer because if she pushes too much the head will swell and we won't be able to get a good grip" says the nurse.

After many hours, time is suddenly of the essence. I look at Donae trying to stay present but my body is so tired I can hardly stand up. Gulping my tea, I give my face a slap trying to wake myself up. I splash tea down my front in my hurry to finish it.

The nurse explains the vacuum extraction method to Donae. They tell her that they can only attempt it three times before deciding on a caesarean. They say this is because of an increased rate of brain damage from more than three pulls on the baby's head.

Donae turns to me. Her face is a blur. From her expression I guess what she is thinking: This is likely to be the last option she has for a vaginal delivery. I squeeze her hand, letting her know I'm with her, whatever she decides.

She tells the nurses she wants to try the vacuum.

The room fills with people and equipment. They are prepping for the birth. The doctor removes the lower half of the bed and puts on gloves and scrubs. Then she lowers a plastic mask over her eyes. "In case of spray," she says when I look at her.

"Are you ready?" she asks.

Donae gulps and brushes back tears. She is utterly exhausted. We are approaching thirty-eight hours on the labor ward. I look at Rafa and we manage a brief smile to each other. I hold Donae's hand, saying silent prayers in my head. She has worked so hard to get to this point. The vacuum cup is placed on the baby's head. Donae heaves and screams loudly as she pushes but the baby doesn't budge. She falls back on the bed panting heavily. First attempt.

My heart is pounding hard. The lights glare down on our tired bodies. I'm in that place of tiredness where things don't seem quite real. But I remind myself that they are and every moment is absolutely crucial. The second push begins. I help her roll up and she bears down hard, grunting. But again, nothing. My eyelids feel like they are on fire. I try to shut out the noise of the room and just focus my attention on Donae. I gently touch my hand to her head getting her attention. We lock eyes and for a moment the noise seems to fall away. There is nothing but Donae and I and the importance of this final push ahead of her.

"Donae, now is the time to talk to baby. Tell baby you must work together for this final push. You can do this. You can both do this. You are incredibly strong." She nods and closes her eyes. I can see she is making the connection.

The final push. We all know this is the last chance for a vaginal delivery. I look at the nurses and her husband. Donae's eyes remain closed as she prepares for this crucial moment. She bears down and the doctor starts the suction. The moment where before she fell back on the bed comes and goes, and she keeps going. Somehow, somewhere she finds the strength to keep pushing. She is awe-inspiring in her strength. My heart is bursting with nerves and pride. The head is crowning and then the head is out! I realize I'm holding my breath and gulp down air to keep going.

The doctor works her hands around the baby's head and then maneuvers the shoulders. First one, then the other. The baby seems to be stuck halfway out for what feels like an age but I'm sure is just a few seconds. Then suddenly the baby is out! The room gasps in relief and amazement. The doctor flips baby onto Donae's chest, and I laugh and cry out from exhaustion and love for the immense strength of this birthing woman. Countless hours of hard labor and she is finally holding her baby. Triumphant!

Donae grabs my arm and tears are running down her face. Her touch says it all. She kisses and cradles her baby smiling with pride. Her husband is next to her. He strokes her hair softly and then kisses their child. I feel my cheeks. They are wet with tears as well. My body begins to shake. I haven't slept for two days and the birth has come in a flood of release. This has been an incredibly hard labor for everyone. I didn't realize how hard I had been working to keep a peaceful environment amidst the tension of fetal distress and threats of surgery.

In letting go, a rush of emotion surges through my body. I have to leave the room and I stumble out, wandering in a trembling daze around the ward. In all this time I have forgotten to take care of myself and have worn myself down to the verge of collapse. I try to steady my breathing but my body just won't cooperate. "You need to sleep!" my brain screams.

Gathering the last of my strength, I step back inside. The birth team are still there. Donae is getting stitches and the baby is being weighed and measured. I walk over to the bed. Donae squeezes my hand. Her facial expression lets me know it's OK to go home. We don't need any words. We both understand what just happened and how deeply we have connected during this birth. I kiss the baby and hug Donae and Rafa one last time. Once again I am reminded that those who give birth are truly warriors.

Oliver *was born at home in Northern California.*

We are one week past Marina's "due date" and protocol dictates we get a non-stress test to check the health of the baby. This has to be done at the hospital even though Marina plans to deliver at home. At the hospital, we announce ourselves to the receptionist when we arrive and then take our seats in the waiting room. We seem to be the only ones around and after a few minutes we are taken down the hall to the delivery ward. The nurse motions for Marina to lie on the bed and then starts hooking her up to the machines.

"We are going to have to stay put until we see at least two accelerations in the baby's heartbeat. We want to check that baby is still active and healthy," she says smiling.

Marina lies on the bed for a few minutes but the baby seems to be sleeping. No accelerations.

"Sometimes when I drink water the baby moves around more." She takes a big gulp from her water bottle.

The monitors sound out the steady *thump thump thump* of the baby's heart and the machine continues to print the report of contractions, producing a little graph of peaks and dips. The nurse looks at the paper.

"Ooh, it looks like you're having some medium-strength contractions right there. Do you feel that?"

"I've been a bit crampy this morning but they haven't been in the usual place. They are lower down," she says, rubbing her hands on the bottom of her belly.

"Those were Braxton Hicks contractions that you've been feeling higher up. These are labor contractions. They seem to in a fairly regular pattern as well. I think you might have this baby tonight. Do you mind if I check you?"

She puts a glove on, lubes her hand and reaches in. "You're four or five centimeters dilated," she says all matter-of-fact.

As she walks out she reminds us we need to see "accels" before we can go. Chad steps out to call the midwife. Things are happening.

Marina looks at me. "I feel nauseous," she says.

Just in time, I grab the trashcan and thrust it towards her. She brings up the water and nuts we just made her eat. The contractions must be getting stronger. Coming back in, the nurse notes two accels and smiles contently.

"Good. Now there is a little bloody show. This is normal and will happen until the baby is born. You are free to go home and have this baby. My guess is before midnight. You can take that bucket with you. For the vomit."

Ripping the paper from the machine, she laughs gently and leaves the room.

"Let's go home and have a baby!" we say together.

As soon as we get home the atmosphere of the house shifts dramatically. It's not a frantic shift, just a simple and direct realization: Marina will birth her baby today. As the reality of this sinks in, a focus descends. Marina goes into her room and begins listening to her hypnobirthing recording. She has been listening and practicing this technique of self-hypnosis, breath, and visualization throughout her pregnancy. Now the time has come put it to use. This transition seems flawless as she gently rocks on her birthing ball, guiding herself into the first stage of her birthing journey. With the sun shining on her and the weather warm and fresh, she looks radiant and serene.

Chad gently runs his fingers up her back and down across her arms. They are settling into their own rhythm. When Marina feels a surge she simply says "push" to Chad and he pushes his palms into the small of her back. She thanks him after every contraction.

Leaving them to their own deepening connection I go outside and pick flowers filling the house with blooms of mid-summer. I hear a car pull up. The first of the birth team has arrived! It's Dianne, Marina mother. I smile, hugging her. Next, Amy the other doula, arrives, followed shortly by Orla the midwife. We head into the house together. The house is com-pletely still with everyone's focus directed towards Marina. Each person quietly sets up their things and settles into the flow of the room. Marina is smoothly guiding herself into a hypnotized state as she works through each contraction. Every surge brings her closer to her baby. Amy keeps repeating, "You are opening." We all hold space and breathe together.

About an hour in, her waters break, gushing clear fluids everywhere. One step closer. It is still light outside and sun is streaming in through the big bay windows. I can hear the roost-ers squawking and the cat slinking around outside wondering what's going on. The changes in the room are subtle, but I can really feel when things start to get more intense. We all seem to be attuned to each other. Marina begins to enter transition, the final and hardest stage of opening before pushing begins. Her strength is truly awe-inspiring. Now and then she moans a deep belly sound from within. She seems to be channeling all of her strength and power downwards. It is all very still.

"I'm going to check you." Orla gloves and reaches inside.

"She is complete," she announces to the room.

Complete. She is fully dilated. The excitement in the room goes up a notch, sending a thrill down my spine. Marina has been moving around a lot as she finds ways to cope with the rapidly intensifying sensations. Visualizing the arrival of her baby she breathes through the surges and sends the energy down to meet the baby. Chad and I both stroke and hold her arms and her legs, rubbing her heels and telling her things like, "That's the way. That's right," in soft, encouraging voices.

The energy we are all holding in the room is so powerful, like we are standing at the edge of something profound and expectant but still unknown. Marina stands up naked and glowing, the sun shining on her. Her eyes are closed and she is gently swaying holding her belly and moaning softly. She appears to be in a deep trance with her baby and her body. No words are spoken.

The clock reads 5:30 p.m. She has been laboring for a little over three hours. We prop her up on pillows and everyone climbs onto the bed or stands around her. Each person offers her counterresistance for her to push against. Orla begins pouring oil over her perineum and stretches her vagina in preparation for the birth.

Just then we hear tires crunching on the gravel and Alice, Marina's best friend, comes running in. She has driven up from San Francisco. There is no time to talk. I gesture for Alice to get on the bed and she falls in place beside her best friend, arms cradling her back as she pushes. What a time to arrive!

Marina gets the hang of it fast. She is making great progress. Alice and I are on the bed behind her rolling her back up as she pushes. We can just make out the tip of the baby's head. A full head of dark brown hair! After each push I place a cold towel on her head as she catches her breath and rests, preparing for the next push. A few more pushes and Orla reaches her hand around the baby's head, maneuvering it gently to make more room for the rest of the body to follow. The head seems enormous to me. I look around. Is anyone else thinking how big this head is? But then suddenly the baby is out! Chad gasps as the baby comes sailing out on a tide of fluids and begins to cry immediately. Wonder! Joy! Awe! He makes good use of his little lungs. His eyes open and he reaches out for his mother. Marina gathers him in her arms, laying him immediately across her chest.

I look around the room and my heart is bursting with joy and pride and honor to be able to witness things like this. Truly there is nothing else like being with a person as they give birth. Marina looks amazing, equal parts awe, shock, and radiant strength. The cord is cut after it stops pulsing. Chad crawls up right next to Marina and nestles the baby to his bare chest, softly singing the words to a song they have been singing to the baby throughout the pregnancy. His voice cracks with emotion. The baby turns at the sound of his voice. Babies are so intelligent. What an honor to be part of this birth, without fear or doubts about the innate abilities of those who carry, nurture, and reproduce life through birth.

HERBS FOR PREGNANCY, BIRTH, AND BEYOND

The People's Medicine

Pregnancy is an excellent time for birth givers, to explore their bodies in depth, to marvel, honor, and celebrate each stage of growth and development and to revel in a heightened sense of awareness, intuition, and deepening sensuality. The body truly undergoes profound changes over the course of pregnancy, doubling its blood volume, adding uterine muscle, amniotic fluid, and a placenta. Add to this the growth of the fetus itself and you begin to realize the true extent of this radical piece of reproductive labor. The effects of these changes can sometimes cause ailments such as morning sickness, mood swings, varicose veins, hemorrhoids, backaches, constipation, and anemia. Many of these symptoms can be soothed and often prevented through the use of medicinal herbs taken alongside a healthy, well-rounded diet.

Working closely with plant medicine throughout pregnancy, birth, and the postpartum period allows us to tap into an ancient system of knowledge that celebrates interdependence and solidarity with the natural environment while supporting avenues for circulating health and healing outside of neoliberal health care systems. When you privatize knowledge about health you foreclose the ability of people to effectively care for themselves and their communities. In reclaiming or "making common" this knowledge we can begin to disrupt this process through demystifying health and bringing medicine back into the hands and hearts of the common people. This ultimately serves as a pathway to greater self-determination and health justice.

Herbal tonics, infusions, poultices, and tinctures have been used throughout the ages in support of all forms of reproductive experience from optimizing fertility and pregnancy to providing contraceptive and abortive care.[17] The following list is by no means exhaustive and interested readers would do well to consultant herbalists, alternative health centers, or one of the many books dedicated to the comprehensive study, identification, preparation, and use of herbs for medicine.[18]

The collection herein is humble in nature and is included as a small taster of what is truly a vast terrain of knowledge for health and healing from the plant world. The intention is to purposefully weave narratives of birth, reproduction, and liberatory politics together with practical knowledge of herbal medicine in order to deepen bonds of solidarity and affinity between the agendas of social justice movements and herbal medicine as a foundation of alternative health care—envisioned here an "act of resistance" to the state monopolization of health. This practical and theoretical knowledge can help move us beyond reliance on patriarchal health care systems, enabling a deeper knowing of our own anatomy and physiology that can help us take charge of our own health. Herbal medicine is part of the common intellect and the original "people's medicine," making it a historically vital part of sustaining and reproducing all grassroots social movements. Let us reclaim and celebrate this ancient wisdom, re-centering it as a key element in the realization of sustainable and cooperative ways of caring for our bodies and our communities.

Herbal Tonics

Herbal tonics have been used by midwives, birth workers, and herbalists for centuries. The unique benefit of tonic herbs lies in their ability to nourish and support the "whole person"—working to nurture physical, spiritual, and mental well-being in a holistic treatment of imbalance. The more tonics are consumed the greater the nourishing effects will be. The following tonics are safe, effective, and time-tested in supporting and nurturing a healthy pregnancy, birth, and postpartum period.

Nettle (*Urtica dioica*)
Parts used: Leaves
Some useful properties: Tonic, nutritive, astringent

Nettle is often thought of as an irritating weed, yet it remains one of the most nourishing tonic herbs available. Nettle provides a rich source of vitamins A, C, D, and K, iron, calcium, potassium, and phosphorous, all of which are essential for maternal and fetal well-being. The high calcium content in nettle helps to reduce cramps and uterine pains, while vitamin K and iron help to strengthen blood, increase hemoglobin, and decrease the likelihood of postpartum hemorrhage. Nettle also supports the kidneys and cleanses the blood supply during pregnancy. The astringent quality of nettle works to tighten and strengthen blood vessels, enabling them to maintain elasticity and thus lessen the likelihood of developing hemorrhoids. This wonderful weed grows abundantly in most wet climates. Go for a walk and harvest some for yourself. It also makes a delicious soup!

Red Raspberry Leaf (*Rubus idaeus*)
Parts used: Leaves
Some useful properties: Tonic, nutritive, astringent

Red raspberry leaf is one of the most widely used uterine and pregnancy herbs. It was originally used by the people of Troy as a female-tonic and fertility aid due to its love-inducing aphrodisiac qualities. It is typically taken as a tea and drunk in the final trimester of pregnancy and postpartum. The plant contains *fragrine*, which is an alkaloid that works to actively

tone and strengthen the muscles of the uterus in preparation
for labor. A toned uterus is able to contract more effectively,
leading to a shortened labor and a decreased risk of miscarriage or postpartum hemorrhage. The plant provides a rich
source of vitamins and minerals including vitamins A, B, C,
and E, iron, calcium, potassium, and phosphorus, which
support a healthy production of milk. Red raspberry leaf continues to be used throughout the world as food, medicine, and
an overall strengthening tonic.

Herbs for Milk Production

There are plenty of plant-based remedies for some of the difficulties that can often accompany nursing. These remedies
offer simple, safe ways for nursing people and their babies to
stay healthy, increase milk supply, and fend off sore nipples.
To keep milk supply flowing freely, try these milk-producing
"galactagogue" herbs. They can be taken as a tea or tincture and
will work best taken in addition to continuing use of nettle and
red raspberry leaf as well as other nutrient- and mineral-rich
herbs such as borage, alfalfa, and red clover. Eating of lots dark
leafy greens, dandelion leaves, and watercress can also be very
beneficial to milk supply.

Fenugreek (*Trigonella foenum-graecum*)
Parts used: Seeds
Some useful properties: Galactagogue, emmenagogue,
digestive

Fenugreek is one of the oldest medicinal herbs in recorded
history. As far back as the Ancient Egyptians it was used to
ease childbirth and increase milk production. Today fenugreek
is still known as a milk-enhancing herb and is probably the
most commonly used galactagogue. It contains the active milk-
producing compound *diosgenin*. It has a distinctive and linger-
ing smell, similar to maple syrup. If you cannot smell this scent
on your skin, you might not be taking enough! Fenugreek can

lower blood sugar levels and should be avoided if you are diabetic or have hypoglycemia. It should also be avoided during pregnancy but is safe to use postpartum.

Goat's Rue (*Galega officinalis*)

Parts used: Leaves

Some useful properties: Galactagogue, emmenagogue, diuretic

Goat's rue is another great herb for stimulating the production of breast milk and has a long usage dating back to the Middle Ages. It has a direct effect on the mammary glands and can actually stimulate further development of breast tissue. It is a good choice for people who have had low milk supply from the early postpartum period. Like fenugreek it can have a lowering effect on blood sugars and should not be used by people with diabetes.

Aromatic Seeds

Parts used: Seeds

Some useful properties: Digestive, galactagogue, carminative

Though not technically galactagogues, aromatic seeds, such as anise, cumin, fennel, caraway, coriander, and dill are excellent aids in supporting plentiful milk supply because they actively stimulate the milk let-down reflex. These seeds are also extremely beneficial to the digestive system. Their soothing effect on the digestive tract is carried through to breast milk, helping to reduce colic and indigestion in breastfeeding babies.

Herbs for Swollen Breasts and Sore Nipples

Painful breasts and nipples are some of the most common problems experienced during nursing. These ailments can inhibit the desire to nurse, which can in turn lead to a decrease in milk production. It is important to treat these complaints as soon as they surface. The best form of treatment is a combination of rest alongside regular hot water soaks and applications of herbal poultices and compresses. Soaking breasts in hot water infused with medicinal herbs or essential oils such as fennel, lavender, and rose, can be incredibly beneficial as hot waters works to relax swollen breast tissues and stimulates circulation for more effective healing. Additionally applying a herbal poultice of fresh or cooked herbs directly onto the breasts, or covering breasts in a cloth soaked in herbal infusion can help to speed recovery enabling feeding to return to normal. Besides herbs, applying cabbage or rhubarb leaves to engorged breasts has also been reported as an effective method for reducing swelling and pain.

Comfrey (*Symphytum officinale*)
Parts used: Leaves
Some useful properties: Anti-inflammatory, astringent, vulnerary

Comfrey has been used to treat wounds and broken bones for centuries. Its name *Symphytum*, comes from the Greek meaning "to grow together." It is famed for its ability to rapidly stimulate new cell growth. When applied as a poultice or compress to painful breasts comfrey soothes irritated and tender breast tissue and reduces inflammation of swollen or engorged breasts. It also helps to reopen clogged milk ducts, allowing breastfeeding to continue. As a compress or soak, comfrey combines well with yarrow and slippery elm to help to draw out further infection. An ointment of comfrey, calendula, and chickweed also works to soothe cracked nipples.

Yarrow (*Achillea millefolium*)
Parts used: Leaves and flowers
Some useful properties: Antiseptic, diaphoretic, analgesic

Yarrow gets its name from the Greek hero Achilles, who is said to have used it to successfully disinfect the wounds of his soldiers in battle. This herb has an analgesic effect, which means it provides almost instantaneous pain relief when applied to engorged breasts or cracked nipples. It is an excellent antiseptic for wounds as it helps to draw out infection and prevents further spreading. If a more prolonged or feverish infection does develop yarrow can be liberally drunk as a tea, together with elderflower, to help break the fever. Yarrow should not be used during pregnancy.

Herbs to Combat Stress and Nourish Vitality

Being pregnant, giving birth, and raising kids isn't always a walk in the park.

If you are consistently feeling worn-down from the stresses that can arise with new parenthood these herbs can help support you in building and maintaining resilience. As nervous system relaxants, these herbs also work to reduce stress levels and improve sleep, enabling an essential and regenerative boost to the body's vital energies. Just what's needed with newborns! These herbs will work best integrated into a nourishing diet rich in magnesium, zinc, B vitamins, and essential fatty acids.

Lemon Balm (*Melissa officinalis*)
Parts used: Stalks and leaves
Some useful properties: Tonic, nervine, antidepressant

Lemon balm has been cultivated in the Mediterranean for around two thousand years and was dedicated to the goddess Diana by the Greeks. Its Latin *Melissa* derives from the Greek word for "bee," so named for its ability to attract bees to the garden. Lemon balm's key medicinal properties are its ability to uplift the spirits, dispel melancholy, and bring overall calm and soothing to the nerves. It is a great herb for postpartum as it works to stabilize mood swings that can be common in the early days of parenthood. Lemon balm is also effective in supporting the release of grief related to sexual trauma and can provide excellent support in processing challenging birth experiences. This herb is soothing and relaxing without causing tiredness. Combines well with motherwort and borage to further reduce anxiety.

Oats (*Avena sativa*)
Parts used: Stalks, leaves, and milky tops
Some useful properties: Tonic, nervine, antidepressant

Both the milky tops and straw of oats have long-term use as a medicine in the treatment of nervous system complaints such as migraines, anxiety, depression, and fatigue. This plant has a nourishing and strengthening effect on the entire nervous system and is especially useful for frayed nerves. A tea or tincture made from the fresh milky tops can effectively support stress management and aid clarity, allowing the mind, body, and spirit to stay calm and centered among the whirlwind of newborns. Oat straw is also uplifting to the spirits and psyche. Although its relaxing effects are immediate, as a tonic herb its long-lasting actions will develop best over time. Nourishment will only grow stronger with consistent use. Combines well with lavender, hops, and chamomile to calm the nerves and aid sleep.

Skullcap (*Scutellaria lateriflora*)
Parts Used: Leaves and flowers
Some useful properties: Nervine, tonic, sedative, anti-spasmodic

Skullcap is a powerful nervine herb native to North America. It is used to support and strengthen the nervous system through increasing resilience to external and internal stressors. Use of skullcap dates back to the first nations of the Americas who used it for female health and menstrual ceremonies. Skullcap is also extremely useful for relieving nerve pain, anxiety, and tension headaches and aiding sleep without causing drowsiness—essential for the body to replenish, regenerate, and cope with life's trials. Combines well with other uplifting herbs such as linden flowers and passionflower. Skullcap should avoided in pregnancy.

Borage (*Borago officinalis*)
Parts Used: Leaves and flowers
Some useful properties: Tonic, nutritive, galactagogue

Borage, a native of the Mediterranean, is a striking plant also known as "starflower" for its memorable blue star-like flowers. It is cultivated in both Europe and the U.S. for its medicinal properties and as a culinary treat—it makes a tasty and beautiful addition to salads! Its usage as medicine dates back at least as far as Romans who are said to have drunk borage tea to fortify themselves for battle. This is probably due to its high nutrient content and essential fatty acids that are vital for health and well-being as well as balancing the emotions. As a tonic herb borage has an especially beneficial effect on the restoring adrenal glands and preventing adrenal fatigue as the result of ongoing stress. This in turn has an overall calming effect through uplifting the spirits and regulating mood swings. Combines well with all the nervine tonic herbs noted above as well as rose and St. John's wort.

An End and a Beginning

Where profit-driven health care meets institutionalized oppression, we experience again and again intrusions that attempt to dictate how birth givers should or should not experience their sexual and reproductive bodies. It is also at these intersections that the value and power of adequate and appropriate care becomes so essential. As we take a step forward, we might ask: how can we collectively reimagine the trajectory of our reproductive experiences as well as the care that unfolds around these experiences? Only when our whole selves are recognized and honored in the care we receive can we come closer to obtaining birth justice—for true reproductive freedom means celebrating the needs of every person at all stages of sexual and reproductive life, not subsuming all bodies within one paradigm of reproductive care. The task of activist birth work is to uphold and further a culture of support in which all people feel they can access appropriate care for the full spectrum of their reproductive needs. In so doing, we can support many ways of birthing, parenting, caregiving, and creating families today. Envisioning birth work as part of a self-reproducing movement—that makes no separation between its political work and the work done in service of reproductive experiences of all kinds—positions birth workers as potentially vital political mediators within intersectional struggles for freedom and dignity. Here, activist birth work joins with larger liberatory movements in centralizing the voices of the historically marginalized while at the same time dismantling systems that seek to control and regulate all forms of human experience. The activist birth worker, co-facilitator of birth and radical caregiver, holds the potential to bring new resonance to these essential struggles and in so doing illuminates the vital connections between birth, body-autonomy, and liberatory justice throughout society.

We birth as we live.

A POLITICAL DICTIONARY

Terms, Concepts, and Organizations

Bay Area Doula Project A collective of doulas that work to increase access to nonjudgmental doula care for a full spectrum of reproductive experiences with a particular focus on abortion care. The collective trains and educates doulas to become full spectrum birth workers. BADP is partnered with ACCESS Women's Health Justice to provide ongoing volunteer support for those seeking abortions.

Birth Giver A person who nurtures other beings inside them and who gives birth. Birth givers may self-identify as women or any number of other genders.

Birth Justice Project A collective of doulas that offer birth support and reproductive health education to incarcerated and formerly incarcerated people from the San Francisco County Jail. BJP also works in partnership with Black Women Birthing Justice and the East Bay Community Support Birth Project to train people color and formerly incarcerated people to become doulas.

Birth Story The story of one's own or someone else's birth. Though hard to recall, one's birth is understood to be one of the most memorable and impressionable experiences of a person's life. Many view reconnecting with one's birth story as a way to shed light on personal behaviors enabling people to better understand themselves and the power of the birthing process as a whole. Knowing one's story is also a necessary step towards transforming one's story.

Birth Worker A caregiver and advocate that supports birth givers to navigate the struggles and triumphs of their reproductive experiences. See also *Certified Nurse Midwife, Certified Professional Midwife, Doula.*

Black Women Birthing Justice A collective of African American, African, Caribbean, and multiracial birth workers working to transform birth experiences for black communities. BWBJ aims to rebuild confidence in giving birth naturally while decreasing the medical violence experienced by black women and other birthing people of color in the United States.

Care Work The frequently "invisiblized" and chronically undervalued labor that is necessary to the reproduction of life and to the continuation and growth of the capitalist market. Care work remains essential to the continuation of societal functioning through providing the nourishment and support necessary to sustain and reproduce the individual and the community anew each day. See also *Reproductive Labor.*

Certified Nurse Midwife A reproductive health care practitioner trained as a nurse with a specialization in maternal health and midwifery. All CNMs are registered and licensed nurses and are primarily trained to work in hospital settings.

Certified Professional Midwife A reproductive health care practitioner trained through the apprenticeship model at an independent midwifery school. The majority of CPMs are trained to deliver babies at home or in freestanding birth centers and are not licensed to practice in the hospital. CPMs are highly regulated by the State and are under constant threat of becoming illegal.

Commons A concept that describes a new form of social relation or a society sustained and reproduced through the direct participation of all reproductive communities. Actions follow a logic opposed to capitalist modes of relating such as mutual aid, cooperation, respect for all beings, and widespread sharing of knowledge and resources. "Commoning" includes consciously creating alternatives to life under capitalism through elaborating more autonomous forms of social reproduction, including the way we collectively "do" birth.

Community A quality of relation that engenders feelings of connection enabling networks of collectivized care to develop that weave people together for a common purpose. Can be used tactfully to rally and unite people as well as to delineate territory that shuts others out. See also *Commons*.

Domestic Worker A person often referred to as a "nanny" or "housekeeper" who performs many of the tasks necessary to sustaining the functioning of *someone else's* family. Typically employed by households so that both parents can continue to participate in the capitalist market. Many women have been able to enter the workforce and break with "traditional" roles expected of them only as a result of employing (and frequently exploiting) domestic workers—who are almost always other women—to perform these tasks for them. A highly underpaid and undervalued job sector. See also *Reproductive Labor*.

Doula *Birth:* A guardian of transitions, gatekeeper, advocate and caregiver. Involves the cultivation and co-creation of an environment free from fear, in which all birth givers feel respected and loved, allowing them to discover their own inner strength as they navigate the dance of labor and emerge into embodied and grounded parenthood.
Postpartum: A mediator, educator, domestic worker and caregiver. Involves supporting new parents and their babies for

the first few months after birth. May include some amount of domestic labor as well as psychological and lactation support for parents as they adjust to new tasks and family dynamics. *Full Spectrum:* An activist, ally and radical caregiver. Involves support for all reproductive experiences and outcomes including, menstruation, birth, abortion, rape, stillbirth, miscarriage, or adoption. Often linked to larger liberatory and intersectional political projects that critically engage the effects of sexuality, race, class, ability, citizenship, and gender-based discrimination on the unfolding of reproductive care.

Doula Salon An educational and social gathering of doulas and birth workers intended to enrich and expand their practice. There is no official "doula school"; education and learning happens informally through collective organizing, skill-sharing, and mentorship. A doula salon provides a space for such co-learning to happen.

Doulas of North America DONA is an international nonprofit educational organization of doulas and educators that oversees and provides certification and accreditation to the vast majority of doula training programs in the country. It is the oldest and largest association of doulas in the world.

East Bay Community Support Birth Project Collaborative project of birth workers that focuses on providing support, mentorship, and doula training to formerly incarcerated communities and communities of color.

Feminism A desire to live and to thrive in a world held in common, where the reproduction of all bodies and all forms of social life are carried out with dignity and respect and where pleasure and sensuality nourish and enrich a spirit of mutual caregiving.

Herbal Medicine The original "people's medicine" that has historically been the means of survival for the dispossessed. Reclaiming knowledge of herbal medicine is often configured within political efforts to demystify health, circulating knowledge of healing outside of and beyond formal institutions that seek to monopolize this knowledge. An emphasis is placed on bringing healing back into the hands, hearts, and bodies of the common people. Includes great respect and mentorship from elders as well as a practice of cooperative earth relations.

Imposter Syndrome A nasty and frequently false premonition that takes hold in the mind and attempts to convince a person that they are not adequate or qualified enough to be performing a particular task, for example birth work. Often the result of working in an environment dominated by men or a majority of white people.

Medical Model of Birth The standard model of care in hospitals today. Labor is conceived as a physical process that can be effectively managed and sped up by medical interventions, which are viewed as vital to the progress of birth. In this framework a strong emphasis is placed on monitoring and recording progress in order to dictate the speed at which labor must unfold.

Natural Model Birth Typically refers to an unmedicated birth in which no labor-augmenting drugs or pain-relieving interventions are used. Tends to place the women, and those who give birth, at the center of care, trusting in their innate abilities to give birth. Labor is usually allowed to progress on its own with as little interference or disruption as possible. Can have a strong spiritual component, conceiving of birth as a major rite of passage that profoundly affect peoples lives. Can be problematically applied when juxtaposed against "medicalized birth" and configured within a language of "choice" or when used to boast; as in "I did it completely *natural*," which has the effect of shaming those who do not or cannot participate for any number of reasons, chosen or not.

Politics An ominous force that is embedded within all cracks and crevasses of social life and all forms of social relation. Has been tactfully presented as existing only in the so-called public sphere in order to maintain structures of dominance and depoliticize the struggles of "private" life, especially reproductive labor and care work.

Pregnancy A time to revel in the exquisite beauty of one's transforming body and find new and inventive ways to have sex. Also a time when it's OK to hurl in a backpack on the bus or eat pickles with jam at 3:00 a.m.

Reproductive Justice Theoretical and activist model that expands the "rights" discourse of reproductive organizing to include an intersectional analysis that addresses the complete physical, mental, spiritual, political, social, environmental, and economic well being of reproducing communities. Grew out of the mobilization of women of color in response to the domination of white middle-class interests in reproductive organizing. Includes the fight for safe and accessible reproductive health care regardless of race, class, gender, sexual orientation, age, or personal history—this means honoring choices to have or *not* have children. Reproductive justice argues that no discussion of "rights" can happen without first addressing the effects of racial, economic, cultural, and structural forms of oppression in which rights are embedded and exercised by different communities.

Reproductive Labor Essential yet frequently unacknowledged and unpaid work that functions as a necessary precursor to all forms of capitalist production, e.g., cooking, cleaning, sex, intimacy, emotional support, and childcare. Also refers to the physical labor of reproducing another human being in and through the act of birthing.

San Francisco General Hospital (SFGH) Doula Program A volunteer shift-based doula program that provides both birth and postpartum doula support to patients at the SFGH.

Self-Reproducing Movement A movement that brings the personal and political together, collapsing the distinction between political work and the work necessary to the reproduction of life itself including the way we "reproduce" ourselves, and others through birth.

SQUAT Birth Journal A quarterly radical midwifery and birth publication that showcases the activism of birth workers involved in Reproductive Justice organizing and full spectrum care. Also highlights activism that expands the boundaries of birth work and what it means to work a radical birth worker today. The journal's retirement was announced in 2015.

White Volunteerism The tendency for white people from privileged backgrounds to think they know what's best for other communities, especially communities of color. Frequently results in unsolicited advice or unwelcome intervention in which white people attempt to speak for others and to implement their own version of "justice."

Organizations Mentioned in This Anthology

Bay Area Doula Project: bayareadoulaproject.org
Birth Justice Project: birthjusticeproject.org
BirthKeepers: birthkeepersummit.com
Black Women Birthing Justice:
    www.blackwomenbirthingjustice.org
Doulas of North America (DONA): www.dona.org
Ecobirth: ecobirth.blogspot.com
Forward Together: forwardtogether.org (previously Asian
    Communities for Reproductive Justice)
Radical Doula: radicaldoula.com
San Francisco General Hospital Doulas: www.sfghdoulas.org/
Sister Song sistersong.net

Further Online Resources

Birth Anarchy: birthanarchy.com
Milk Junkies: www.milkjunkies.net
Our Bodies Ourselves www.ourbodiesourselves.org/
Planned Parenthood: www.plannedparenthood.org/
RH Reality Check: rhrealitycheck.org/
The Doula Project: www.doulaproject.org
Through the Looking Glass: www.lookingglass.org/
Trans Birth: www.transbirth.com

Bibliography

Anzaldúa, Gloria. *Borderlands/La Frontera: The New Mestiza*. San Francisco: Aunt Lute Books, 1987.

Block, Jennifer. *Pushed: The Painful Truth about Childbirth and Modern Maternity Care*. Cambridge, MA: Da Capo Press: 2007.

Boston Women's Health Book Collective. *Our Bodies, Ourselves*. New York: Simon & Schuster, 2011.

Chrisler, Joan C., ed. *Reproductive Justice: A Global Concern*. Santa Barbara, CA: Praeger Publishers, 2012.

Collins, Patricia Hill. *Black Feminist Thought: Knowledge, Consciousness, and the Politics of Empowerment*. New York: Routledge, 2000.

Dalla Costa, Mariarosa, and Selma James. *The Power of Women and the Subversion of the Community*. Bristol: Falling Wall Press, 1975.

Davis-Floyd, Robbie. *Birth as an American Rite of Passage*. 2nd ed. Berkeley: University of California Press, 2003.

Ehrenreich, Barbara, and Deirdre English. *Witches, Midwives, and Nurses: A History of Women Healers*. 2nd ed. New York: Feminist Press, 2010.

Federation of Feminist Women's Health Centers. *A New View of a Woman's Body*. New York: Simon & Schuster, 1981.

Federici, Silvia. *Caliban and the Witch: Women, the Body and Primitive Accumulation*. New York: Autonomedia, 2004.

———. *Revolution at Point Zero: Housework, Reproduction, and Feminist Struggle*. Oakland: PM Press, 2012.

Flavin, Jeanne, *Our Bodies, Our Crimes: The Policing of Women's Reproduction in America*. New York: NYU Press, 2009.

Gaskin, Ina May. *Spiritual Midwifery*. 4th ed. Summertown, TN: Book Publishing Company, 2002.

———. *Ina May's Guide to Childbirth*. New York: Bantam Books, 2003.

———. *Birth Matters: A Midwife's Manifesto*. New York: Seven Stories Press, 2011.

Gladstar, Rosemary. *Herbal Healing for Women*. Boston: Touchstone, 1993.

———. *Herbs for Common Ailments: How to Make and Use Herbal Remedies for Home Health Care*. North Adams, MA: Storey Publishing, 2014.

Gonzales, Patrisia. *Red Medicine: Traditional Indigenous Rites of Birthing and Healing*. Tucson: University of Arizona Press, 2012.

Green, James. *The Herbal Medicine-Maker's Handbook: A Home Manual*. New York: Crossing Press, 2000.

Grieve, Maud. *A Modern Herbal*. Mineola, NY: Dover Publications, 1972.

Gurr, Barbara. *Reproductive Justice: The Politics of Health Care for Native American Women*. New Brunswick, NJ: Rutgers University Press, 2014.

Hoffman, David. *Holistic Herbal: A Safe and Practical Guide to Making and Using Herbal Remedies*. London: Thorsons, 2002.

hooks, bell. *Talking Back: Thinking Feminist, Thinking Black*. New York: Routledge, 2014.

Kitzinger, Sheila. *Your Baby, Your Way*. New York: Pantheon, 1987.

———. *Rediscovering Birth*, New York: Pocket Books, 2000.

———. *The Complete Book of Pregnancy and Childbirth*. 4th ed. New York: Alfred. A. Knopf, 2003.

Law, Victoria, and China Martens. *Don't Leave Your Friends Behind: Concrete Ways to Support Families in Social Justice Movements and Communities*. Oakland: PM Press, 2012.

Lorde, Audre. *Sister Outsider*. Berkeley: Crossing Press, 2007.

Morgen, Sandra. *Into Our Own Hands: The Women's Health Movement in the United States, 1969–1990*. New Brunswick, NJ: Rutgers University Press, 2002.

Oparah, Julia Chinyere, and Alicia. D. Bonaparte. *Birthing Justice: Black Women, Pregnancy, and Childbirth*. London: Routledge, 2015.

Pérez, Miriam Z. *The Radical Doula Guide: A Political Primer for Full Spectrum Pregnancy and Childbirth Support*. Self-published, 2012.

Roberts, Dorothy. *Killing the Black Body: Race, Reproduction, and the Meaning of Liberty*. New York: Vintage Books, 1997.

Romm, Aviva. J. *The Natural Pregnancy Book: Herbs, Nutrition, and Other Holistic Choices*. Berkeley: Celestial Arts, 2003.

Schiller, Rebecca. *All That Matters,* London: The Guardian Shorts, 2015.

Silliman, Jael, Marlene Gerber Fried, Loretta. J. Ross, and Elena Gutiérrez. *Undivided Rights: Women of Color Organize for Reproductive Justice.* Boston: South End Press, 2004.

Simkin, Penny, and Phyllis Klaus. *When Survivors Give Birth: Understanding and Healing the Effects of Early Sexual Abuse on Childbearing Women.* Seattle: Class Day Publishing, 2004.

Weed, Susun. *Wise Women Herbal for the Childbearing Year.* New York: Ash Tree Publishing, 1996.

About the Authors

Alana Apfel is a birth worker, writer, and community gardener. She is a graduate of the Anthropology and Social Change program of the California Institute of Integral Studies. As a birth justice activist she has been involved with the San Francisco General Hospital Doula Program, BirthWays community education center in Berkeley, and the growing international BirthKeepers coalition. She now lives and works in Bristol, UK, where she is part of the Positive Birth Movement and is training to be a midwife in the National Health Service. This is her first book.

Loretta J. Ross was a cofounder and National Coordinator of the SisterSong Women of Color Reproductive Justice Collective. She is one of the creators of the term "Reproductive Justice," coined by African American women following the International Conference on Population and Development in Cairo.

Victoria Law is a mother, photographer, and writer. She is the author of *Resistance Behind Bars: The Struggles of Incarcerated Women* and coeditor of *Don't Leave Your Friends Behind: Concrete Ways to Support Families in Social Justice Movements and Communities.*

Silvia Federici is a feminist activist, writer, and teacher. In 1972 she was one of the cofounders of the International

Feminist Collective, the organization that launched the international campaign for Wages for Housework. In the 1990s, after a period of teaching and research in Nigeria, she was active in the anti-globalization movement and the U.S. anti-death penalty movement. She is the author of *Revolution at Point Zero: Housework, Reproduction, and Feminist Struggle*.

Notes

1   Lara N. Dotson-Renta, "Raising a Biracial Child as a Mother of Color," *The Atlantic*, September 19, 2015, http://www.theatlantic.com/ politics/archive/2015/09/raising-a-biracial-child-as-a-mother-of-color/405739/ and Eisa Nefertari Ulen, "Black Parenting Matters: Raising Children in a World of Police Terror," *Truthout*, October 1, 2015, http://www.truth-out.org/opinion/item/33040-black-parenting-matters-raising-children-in-a-world-of-police-terror.

2   Asian Communities for Reproductive Justice, "What Is Reproductive Justice?" http://strongfamiliesmovement.org/ what-is-reproductive-justice.

3   Mariarosa Dalla Costa and Selma James, *The Power of Women and the Subversion of the Community* (Bristol: Falling Wall Press Ltd., 1975). See also Selma James's 2012 interview on *Democracy Now!* http://www.democracynow.org/2012/4/16/housework_as_work_ selma_james/ and the Global Women's Strike website, http://www. globalwomenstrike.net/.

4   Victoria Law, "U.S. Prisons and Jails Are Threatening the Lives of Pregnant Women and Babies," *In These Times*, September 28, 2015, http://inthesetimes.com/article/18410.

5   Silvia Federici, *Revolution at Point Zero: Housework, Reproduction, and Feminist Struggle* (Oakland: PM Press, 2012), 147.

6   Audre Lorde, *Sister Outsider: Essays and Speeches* (Berkeley: Crossing Press, 2007), 138.

7   See on this topic Maria Mies, *Patriarchy and Accumulation on a World Scale: Women in the International Division of Labour* (New York: Zed Books Ltd., 1998) and Federici, *Revolution at Point Zero*.

8   Federici, *Revolution at Point Zero*, 122.

9   See on this topic the anthology *Undivided Rights: Women of Color Organize for Reproductive Justice*, edited by Jael Silliman, Marlene Gerber Fried, Loretta J. Ross, and Elena Gutiérrez (Boston: South End Press, 2004); Joan C. Chrisler, ed., *Reproductive Justice: A*

Global Concern (Santa Barbara, CA: Praeger Publishers, 2012); and Dorothy Roberts, *Killing the Black Body: Race, Reproduction and the Meaning of Liberty* (New York: Vintage Books, 1997) for examples of reproductive activism that address the lived experience of communities of color from an intersectional human rights perspective. For current organizing and action, see also the collective work of SisterSong, http://sistersong.net/ and Forward Together, http://forwardtogether.org/.

10 Scopolamine, known as the "twilight sleep" drug when administered in combination with morphine, was routinely used by doctors till the 1960s to render women unconscious during the birth of their children in hospital.

11 For examples from the early years of the "childbirth revival," see the selected works of Ina May Gaskin, the most famous and influential being *Spiritual Midwifery*, 4th ed. (Summertown: Book Publishing Company, 2002 [1975]). See also the selected works of anthropologist Sheila Kitzinger, whose early work includes *The Complete Book of Pregnancy and Childbirth* (New York: Alfred A. Knopf, 2003 [1980]) and *Your Baby, Your Way* (New York: Pantheon, 1987). For more in-depth information on the topic of women's sexuality and health more generally, see the Boston Women's Health Book Collective, *Our Bodies, Ourselves* (New York: Simon & Schuster, 2011), and the Federation of Feminist Women's Health Centers, *A New View of a Woman's Body* (New York: Simon & Schuster, 1981). The women's health movement, like feminism as a whole, has faced ideological and political struggles in addressing the effects of racism and classism on movement-building, coalitions, representation, and the possibilities and limits of collective action and identity. For an overview of the history and challenges of the women's health movement during this time, see Sandra Morgen, *Into Our Own Hands: The Women's Health Movement in the United States, 1969–1990* (New Brunswick, NJ: Rutgers University Press, 2002). From the 1980s onwards critical scholarship on feminism, particularly by women of color, served to radically reconfigured and call into question the language and nature of feminist practice, such as: bell hooks, *Talking Back: Thinking Feminist, Thinking Black* (New York: Routledge, 2014 [1989]); Audre Lorde, *Sister Outsider: Essays and Speeches* (Berkeley: Crossing Press, 2007); Chandra Talpade Mohanty, *Feminism Without Borders: Decolonizing Theory, Practicing Solidarity* (Durham: Duke University Press, 2003); and Patricia Hill Collins, *Black Feminist Thought: Knowledge, Consciousness, and the Politics of*

Empowerment (New York: Routledge, 2000). In examining the problems of formulating a "universality" of gender oppression they sought to draw attention to the dangerous invisibilization of categories of race and class that often occur in relation to gender. Here the necessity of historicizing and politically situating both difference and resistance is stressed in order to support an intersectional movement for the rights of women based on the *particularities* of oppression experienced between different communities. Definitions of political agency or autonomy may necessarily materialize in different ways in this framing yet affinity to a common movement for human rights holds true throughout. This scholarship has radically redefined the nature and language of birth and reproductive activism, resulting in a diversifying and expanding movement that is explored in this text.

12 See Jeanne Flavin, *Our Bodies, Our Crimes: The Policing of Women's Reproduction in America* (New York: NYU Press, 2009) for a powerful examination into how different bodies are either validated or invalidated by the criminal justice system as acceptable to "reproduce," make autonomous decisions, have economic freedom, and parent their children.

13 For an analysis of ongoing health inequities in U.S. maternity care, see Dorothy Roberts, *Killing the Black Body: Race, Reproduction and the Meaning of Liberty* (New York: Vintage Books, 1997), and Jennifer Block, *Pushed: The Painful Truth about Childbirth and Modern Maternity Care* (Cambridge, MA: Da Capo Press, 2007).

14 Christina H. Morton and Elayne G. Clift, *Birth Ambassadors: Doulas and the Re-emergence of Woman-Supported Birth in America* (Amarillo, TX: Praeclarus Press, 2014), 205.

15 Ibid., 204.

16 World Health Organization, "The Prevention and Elimination of Disrespect and Abuse during Facility-Based Childbirth," 2015, http://www.who.int/reproductivehealth/topics/maternal_perinatal/statement-childbirth/en/.

17 See on this topic: Barbara Ehrenreich and Deirdre English, *Witches, Midwives, Nurses: A History of Women Healers* (New York: Feminist Press, 2010); Silvia Federici, *Caliban and the Witch: Women, the Body and Primitive Accumulation* (New York: Autonomedia, 2004); and Patrisia Gonzales, *Red Medicine: Traditional Indigenous Rites of Birthing and Healing* (Tucson: University of Arizona Press, 2012), for a history on the persecution of women's knowledge of herbs and healing, birthing attendants and indigenous healing practices from Europe to the colonial Americas.

18 See on this topic Susun Weed, *Wise Women Herbal for the Childbearing Year* (New York: Ash Tree Publishing, 1996); Anne McIntyre, *Herbs for Pregnancy and Childbirth*; Aviva Romm, *The Natural Pregnancy Book* (Berkeley: Celestial Arts, 2003); and Rosemary Gladstar, *Herbal Healing for Women* (Boston: Touchstone, 1993). For more general herbal medicine guides, see Maud Grieve, *A Modern Herbal* (Mineola, NY: Dover Publications Inc., 1972); David Hoffman, *Holistic Herbal: A Safe and Practical Guide to Making and Using Herbal Remedies* (London: Thorsons, 2002); Rosemary Gladstar, *Herbs for Common Ailments: How to Make and Use Herbal Remedies for Home Health Care* (North Adams, MA: Storey Publishing, 2014); James Green, *The Herbal Medicine-Makers Handbook: A Home Manual* (New York: Crossing Press, 2000).

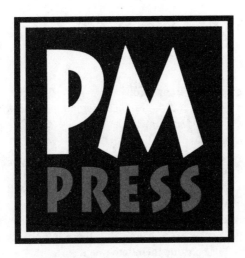

PM Press is an independent, radical publisher of critically
necessary books for our tumultuous times. Our aim is to deliver
bold political ideas and vital stories to all walks of life and arm the
dreamers to demand the impossible. Founded in 2007 by a small
group of people with decades of publishing, media, and organizing
experience, we have sold millions of copies of our books, most
often one at a time, face to face. We're old enough to know what
we're doing and young enough to know what's at stake. Join us to
create a better world.

PM Press
PO Box 23912
Oakland CA 94623
510-703-0327
www.pmpress.org

PM Press in Europe
europe@pmpress.org
www.pmpress.org.uk

FRIENDS OF PM

These are indisputably momentous times—the financial system is melting down globally and the Empire is stumbling. Now more than ever there is a vital need for radical ideas.

In the many years since its founding—and on a mere shoestring—PM Press has risen to the formidable challenge of publishing and distributing knowledge and entertainment for the struggles ahead. With hundreds of releases to date, we have published an impressive and stimulating array of literature, art, music, politics, and culture. Using every available medium, we've succeeded in connecting those hungry for ideas and information to those putting them into practice.

Friends of PM allows you to directly help impact, amplify, and revitalize the discourse and actions of radical writers, filmmakers, and artists. It provides us with a stable foundation from which we can build upon our early successes and provides a much-needed subsidy for the materials that can't necessarily pay their own way. You can help make that happen—and receive every new title automatically delivered to your door once a month—by joining as a Friend of PM Press. And, we'll throw in a free T-shirt when you sign up.

Here are your options:
- **$30 a month** Get all books and pamphlets plus 50% discount on all webstore purchases
- **$40 a month** Get all PM Press releases (including CDs and DVDs) plus 50% discount on all webstore purchases
- **$100 a month** Superstar—Everything plus PM merchandise, free downloads, and 50% discount on all webstore purchases

For those who can't afford $30 or more a month, we have **Sustainer Rates** at $15, $10, and $5. Sustainers get a free PM Press T-shirt and a 50% discount on all purchases from our website.

Your Visa or Mastercard will be billed once a month, until you tell us to stop. Or until our efforts succeed in bringing the revolution around. Or the financial meltdown of Capital makes plastic redundant. Whichever comes first.

In, Against, and Beyond Capitalism: The San Francisco Lectures

John Holloway
with a Preface by Andrej Grubačić

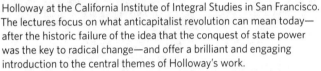

IN, AGAINST, AND BEYOND CAPITALISM

The San Francisco Lectures

JOHN HOLLOWAY

Preface by Andrej Grubačić

ISBN: 978-1-62963-109-7
$14.95   112 pages

In, Against, and Beyond Capitalism is based
on three recent lectures delivered by John
Holloway at the California Institute of Integral Studies in San Francisco.
The lectures focus on what anticapitalist revolution can mean today—
after the historic failure of the idea that the conquest of state power
was the key to radical change—and offer a brilliant and engaging
introduction to the central themes of Holloway's work.

The lectures take as their central challenge the idea that "We Are the
Crisis of Capital and Proud of It." This runs counter to many leftist
assumptions that the capitalists are to blame for the crisis, or that crisis
is simply the expression of the bankruptcy of the system. The only way
to see crisis as the possible threshold to a better world is to understand
the failure of capitalism as the face of the push of our creative force. This
poses a theoretical challenge. The first lecture focuses on the meaning
of "We," the second on the understanding of capital as a system of
social cohesion that systematically frustrates our creative force, and the
third on the proposal that we are the crisis of this system of cohesion.

"His Marxism is premised on another form of logic, one that affirms
movement, instability, and struggle. This is a movement of thought that
affirms the richness of life, particularity (non-identity) and 'walking
in the opposite direction'; walking, that is, away from exploitation,
domination, and classification. Without contradictory thinking
in, against, and beyond the capitalist society, capital once again
becomes a reified object, a thing, and not a social relation that signifies
transformation of a useful and creative activity (doing) into (abstract)
labor. Only open dialectics, a right kind of thinking for the wrong kind
of world, non-unitary thinking without guarantees, is able to assist us in
our contradictory struggle for a world free of contradiction." —Andrej
Grubačić, from his Preface

"Holloway's work is infectiously optimistic."
—Steven Poole, the *Guardian* (UK)

Anthropocene or Capitalocene? Nature, History, and the Crisis of Capitalism

Edited by Jason W. Moore

ISBN: 978-1-62963-148-6

$21.95   304 pages

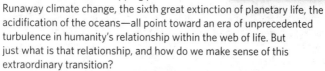

The Earth has reached a tipping point.
Runaway climate change, the sixth great extinction of planetary life, the acidification of the oceans—all point toward an era of unprecedented turbulence in humanity's relationship within the web of life. But just what is that relationship, and how do we make sense of this extraordinary transition?

Anthropocene or Capitalocene? offers answers to these questions from a dynamic group of leading critical scholars. They challenge the theory and history offered by the most significant environmental concept of our times: the Anthropocene. But are we living in the Anthropocene, literally the "Age of Man"? Is a different response more compelling, and better suited to the strange—and often terrifying—times in which we live? The contributors to this book diagnose the problems of Anthropocene thinking and propose an alternative: the global crises of the twenty-first century are rooted in the Capitalocene; not the Age of Man but the Age of Capital.

Anthropocene or Capitalocene? offers a series of provocative essays on nature and power, humanity, and capitalism. Including both well-established voices and younger scholars, the book challenges the conventional practice of dividing historical change and contemporary reality into "Nature" and "Society," demonstrating the possibilities offered by a more nuanced and connective view of human environment-making, joined at every step with and within the biosphere. In distinct registers, the authors frame their discussions within a politics of hope that signal the possibilities for transcending capitalism, broadly understood as a "world-ecology" that joins nature, capital, and power as a historically evolving whole.

Contributors include Jason W. Moore, Eileen Crist, Donna J. Haraway, Justin McBrien, Elmar Altvater, Daniel Hartley, and Christian Parenti.

Revolution at Point Zero: Housework, Reproduction, and Feminist Struggle

Silvia Federici

ISBN: 978-1-60486-333-8
$15.95   208 pages

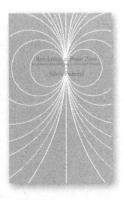

Written between 1974 and 2012, *Revolution at Point Zero* collects forty years of research and theorizing on the nature of housework, social reproduction, and women's struggles on this terrain—to escape it, to better its conditions, to reconstruct it in ways that provide an alternative to capitalist relations.

Indeed, as Federici reveals, behind the capitalist organization of work and the contradictions inherent in "alienated labor" is an explosive ground zero for revolutionary practice upon which are decided the daily realities of our collective reproduction.

Beginning with Federici's organizational work in the Wages for Housework movement, the essays collected here unravel the power and politics of wide but related issues including the international restructuring of reproductive work and its effects on the sexual division of labor, the globalization of care work and sex work, the crisis of elder care, the development of affective labor, and the politics of the commons.

"Finally we have a volume that collects the many essays that over a period of four decades Silvia Federici has written on the question of social reproduction and women's struggles on this terrain. While providing a powerful history of the changes in the organization of reproductive labor, Revolution at Point Zero *documents the development of Federici's thought on some of the most important questions of our time: globalization, gender relations, the construction of new commons."*
—Mariarosa Dalla Costa, coauthor of *The Power of Women and the Subversion of the Community* and *Our Mother Ocean*

Revolutionary Mothering: Love on the Front Lines

Edited by Alexis Pauline Gumbs,
China Martens, and Mai'a Williams
with a preface by Loretta J. Ross

ISBN: 978-1-62963-110-3
$17.95   272 pages

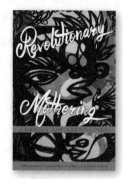

Inspired by the legacy of radical and queer
black feminists of the 1970s and '80s,
Revolutionary Mothering places marginalized mothers of color at the
center of a world of necessary transformation. The challenges we face as
movements working for racial, economic, reproductive, gender, and food
justice, as well as anti-violence, anti-imperialist, and queer liberation
are the same challenges that many mothers face every day. Oppressed
mothers create a generous space for life in the face of life-threatening
limits, activate a powerful vision of the future while navigating tangible
concerns in the present, move beyond individual narratives of choice
toward collective solutions, live for more than ourselves, and remain
accountable to a future that we cannot always see. *Revolutionary
Mothering* is a movement-shifting anthology committed to birthing new
worlds, full of faith and hope for what we can raise up together.

Contributors include June Jordan, Malkia A. Cyril, Esteli Juarez, Cynthia
Dewi Oka, Fabiola Sandoval, Sumayyah Talibah, Victoria Law, Tara
Villalba, Lola Mondragón, Christy NaMee Eriksen, Norma Angelica
Marrun, Vivian Chin, Rachel Broadwater, Autumn Brown, Layne Russell,
Noemi Martinez, Katie Kaput, alba onofrio, Gabriela Sandoval, Cheryl
Boyce Taylor, Ariel Gore, Claire Barrera, Lisa Factora-Borchers, Fabielle
Georges, H. Bindy K. Kang, Terri Nilliasca, Irene Lara, Panquetzani,
Mamas of Color Rising, tk karakashian tunchez, Arielle Julia Brown,
Lindsey Campbell, Micaela Cadena, and Karen Su.

*"This collection is a treat for anyone that sees class and that needs to learn
more about the experiences of women of color (and who doesn't?!). There
is no dogma here, just fresh ideas and women of color taking on capitalism,
anti-racist, anti-sexist theory-building that is rooted in the most primal
of human connections, the making of two people from the body of one:
mothering."*
—Barbara Jensen, author of *Reading Classes: On Culture and Classism in
America*

Don't Leave Your Friends Behind: Concrete Ways to Support Families in Social Justice Movements and Communities

Edited by Victoria Law and
China Martens

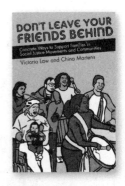

ISBN: 978-1-60486-396-3
$17.95   256 pages

Don't Leave Your Friends Behind is a collection of concrete tips,
suggestions, and narratives on ways that non-parents can support
parents, children, and caregivers in their communities, social
movements, and collective processes. *Don't Leave Your Friends Behind*
focuses on issues affecting children and caregivers within the larger
framework of social justice, mutual aid, and collective liberation.

How do we create new, nonhierarchical structures of support and
mutual aid, and include all ages in the struggle for social justice? There
are many books on parenting, but few on being a good community
member and a good ally to parents, caregivers, and children as we
collectively build a strong all-ages culture of resistance. Any group of
parents will tell you how hard their struggles are and how they are left
out, but no book focuses on how allies can address issues of caretakers'
and children's oppression. Many well-intentioned childless activists
don't interact with young people on a regular basis and don't know how.
Don't Leave Your Friends Behind provides them with the resources and
support to get started.

Contributors include: The Bay Area Childcare Collective, Ramsey Beyer,
Rozalinda Borcilă, Mariah Boone, Marianne Bullock, Lindsey Campbell,
Briana Cavanaugh, CRAP! Collective, a de la maza pérez tamayo, Ingrid
DeLeon, Clayton Dewey, David Gilbert, A.S. Givens, Jason Gonzales,
Tiny (aka Lisa Gray-Garcia), Jessica Hoffman, Heather Jackson, Rahula
Janowski, Sine Hwang Jensen, Agnes Johnson, Simon Knaphus, Victoria
Law, London Pro-Feminist Men's Group, Amariah Love, Oluko Lumumba,
mama raccoon, Mamas of Color Rising/Young Women United, China
Martens, Noemi Martinez, Kathleen McIntyre, Stacey Milbern, Jessica
Mills, Tomas Moniz, Coleen Murphy, Maegan 'la Mamita Mala' Ortiz,
Traci Picard, Amanda Rich, Fabiola Sandoval, Cynthia Ann Schemmer,
Mikaela Shafer, Mustafa Shakur, Kate Shapiro, Jennifer Silverman,
Harriet Moon Smith, Mariahadessa Ekere Tallie, Darran White Tilghman,
Jessica Trimbath, Max Ventura, and Mari Villaluna.

Resistance Behind Bars: The Struggles of Incarcerated Women, 2nd Edition

Victoria Law with an Introduction by Laura Whitehorn

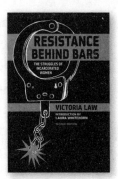

ISBN: 978-1-60486-583-7
$20.00   320 pages

In 1974, women imprisoned at New York's maximum-security prison at Bedford Hills staged what is known as the August Rebellion. Protesting the brutal beating of a fellow prisoner, the women fought off guards, holding seven of them hostage, and took over sections of the prison.

While many have heard of the 1971 Attica prison uprising, the August Rebellion remains relatively unknown even in activist circles. *Resistance Behind Bars* is determined to challenge and change such oversights. As it examines daily struggles against appalling prison conditions and injustices, *Resistance* documents both collective organizing and individual resistance among women incarcerated in the U.S. Emphasizing women's agency in resisting the conditions of their confinement through forming peer education groups, clandestinely arranging ways for children to visit mothers in distant prisons and raising public awareness about their lives, *Resistance* seeks to spark further discussion and research into the lives of incarcerated women and galvanize much-needed outside support for their struggles.

This updated and revised edition of the 2009 PASS Award winning book includes a new chapter about transgender, transsexual, intersex, and gender-variant people in prison.

"Victoria Law's eight years of research and writing, inspired by her unflinching commitment to listen to and support women prisoners, has resulted in an illuminating effort to document the dynamic resistance of incarcerated women in the United States."
—Roxanne Dunbar-Ortiz

"Written in regular English, rather than academese, this is an impressive work of research and reportage"
—Mumia Abu-Jamal, death row political prisoner and author of *Live From Death Row*